CANCER! WHAT NOW?

Essential Steps to Promote Wellness

Robert Dames

CANCER! WHAT NOW?
Essential Steps to Promote Wellness
www.cancerwhatnowbook.com

Paperback ISBN: 979-8334479654

Publisher
10-10-10 Publishing
Markham, ON Canada

Printed in Canada and the United States of America

This book is dedicated to my lovely bride, Beth, who carried and cared for our family during difficult circumstances. Your patience, affirming unconditional love, continues to amaze me.

To our sons Noah, Chris, and Joseph, who have brought me much joy through uncertain times; you are becoming incredible young men.

To friends and family members, your support was stabilizing to our family. And, of course, my amazing little bro, Mike, and your bone marrow stem cells; you literally gave me life. I can't imagine ever being able to repay your love.

Finally, I want to thank all the doctors and nurses who guided me and supported my efforts to claim victory over cancer.

Table of Contents

THE GREATEST ASSET OF A NATION IS THE HEALTH OF ITS PEOPLE.

William J. Mayo, MD
Founder of the Mayo Clinic

NOTE TO READER

BECOMING A VICTOR

This book is a journey of what I learned along a road traveled by nearly 2 million people in the United States alone in 2021. Along the way, I increased my understanding of cancer and other diseases, the importance of how we live, the food we eat, the value of exercise, and how it influences our genes.

Well known by anyone who has endured cancer, either themselves or with a loved one, it is a marathon, not a sprint. Some patients make it to the destination of remission. Unfortunately, others battle with all they have to give, and the enemy still prevails. It is not a fair fight. I hope you will gain a greater possibility of succeeding in your desire to win by reading this book. When I say "WIN," I am referring not only to banishing a disease from your physical body but to not letting it beat you mentally and emotionally, as you ride a roller coaster of emotions.

I have chosen not to refer to myself as a survivor because I believe survivorship connotes being a victim. Victimhood is an attitude of believing there is nothing I can do about it and being at the mercy of the disease and giving in mentally, allowing it to steal away time and energy that is better used for the joy of being with my loved ones, friends, and the experiences of life. A positive mind is essential to empower yourself with a fighting chance against a formidable foe.

The purpose of this book is to share with you what I did and how I did it, and what I have learned. Every desire to achieve an outcome, regardless of what it is, begins with a single light of hope in the darkness. That light may only brighten the path enough to show one step at a time, yet it can give us direction. There are times when advancing in the dark will be necessary, not knowing what lies ahead.

To become healthy, you must learn to act healthfully through your personal efforts. As the story goes, sailing boats can sail in many directions, even when the wind blows in only one direction. Decide to be the captain of your ship, the master of your journey, directing and adjusting your sails as necessary, regardless of the wind.

Thanks for your commitment to reading my story. For those who face the challenge of cancer, I truly hope this book will be a valuable guide and motivator in your journey to win, not just as I have defined it, but as you see it, to assist you in healing physically and empower you to move away from a passive role to a more active one. These habits can improve not just your physical well-being but also your emotional comfort while assisting in developing a new attitude toward life.

"The time is always right to do what is right."
– Dr. Martin Luther King Jr.

FOREWORD

Are you currently dealing with a cancer diagnosis, or do you know someone who is?

Robert Dames, author of *Cancer ... What Now?,* has gone through three cancer diagnoses in ten years. He has considerable experience traveling along the road of ill health. But, never one to let his destiny lie in the hands of fate, he took personal steps to bolster the efforts of the medical experts in the field of oncology/hematology care, to increase the prospects of beating the disease. He has recorded many valuable aspects of this journey, and now you can benefit from his awareness of healthy living habits.

By adopting the material in his book, you have the opportunity to enjoy life more fully, regardless of your condition. As Robert states, these are no magic cures, but there are things you can do to promote a better experience in your battle with cancer, and improve your quality of life.

Robert has laid out a plan for being a warrior against cancer, or for any ailment you may desire to claim victory over. He is determined to have you take control of your health, your life, and your future, and not just let fate decide. He believes life happens for you, and how you handle any experience that comes your way can be empowering or defeating, depending on how you classify each experience in your mind.

Though I am not a medical doctor, I find Robert's book illuminating, and his knowledge of the subject helpful. If you want to enjoy increased health and wellness, especially if you are dealing with cancer, some great advice is accessible to you within the pages that follow.

Please take advantage of the information in this book. But do not just read it. Instead, implement the strategies on these pages and enjoy some impactful results.

Raymond Aaron
New York Times Bestselling Author

Chapter 1

Surprise!

"Life is what happens to us while we are making other plans."
– Allen Saunders

While I lay in my bed on an October morning with my fingers intertwined behind my head, I was daydreaming about the house my wife Beth and I were building and the new baby who was on the way. I reached across my chest with my right hand to scratch under my arm. It was then I noticed a little bump. I thought, is it the same on the other side? I checked my right underarm, and I found no lump. Feeling around the area more intently, I noticed it went deeper into the pit of my arm. It did not hurt, was hard when I squeezed it, and seemed to be about the diameter of a medium-size gum ball.

I reasoned that it was probably a swollen lymph gland since I had recently had a sinus infection, and then I forgot about it. The process of building a new house and my second child coming provided plenty of other things that needed my attention. I was health conscious, felt terrific, had lots of energy, worked out three days a week, ran another three days per week, and was careful about my eating habits, so no worries.

Just after Christmas of 2000, we received a late gift in the likes of the early arrival of our second son Christopher. Our scheduled New Year's Day baby came to us on December 28th in the middle of the night. Perhaps this is why he was our night owl for many years. He is a healthy, happy, and tough kid.

Between my schedule as a pilot, the recent birth of a son, and putting the finishing touches on our new house, I was busy. There was not much time to think about many things other than the tasks at hand each day. I continued my weekly regiments of working out and running. These I find to be beneficial both physically and mentally. Keeping the muscles toned and at working capacity is favorable to denying age with dignity.

As a captain for a commercial airline, I am obligated to have physical examinations every six months with an FAA-qualified and approved doctor. It was not until the following February, during an appointment with my aeromedical physician, the late Dr. Kreyling, who I counted as a friend since we knew each other as pilot comrades before he was my aviation doctor, that the question of this lump under my arm surfaced again.

Toward the close of the exam, we talked about my new son Christopher and my two-year-old son Noah. Then he asked me if everything else was okay. This was an open question, as he was looking to be sure that I was not overly stressed with both my home life and my work. You don't want a distracted pilot flying your airplane, because it leads to mistakes. Initially, I said, "Yes, things are great." Then I remembered the little lump under my arm, and I was not even sure if it was still there. I mentioned it to him, and he took the time to check it out. "How long has it been there?" he asked. I explained to him how I noticed it the previous October. He told me it's probably nothing to worry over. Nonetheless, I should see my regular doctor and get another opinion.

Two weeks later, my primary care physician probed around for a while and came to the same conclusion as Dr. Kreyling: "Probably nothing to worry over. Your health is excellent," followed by, "But let's get a biopsy done to be sure."

A general surgeon extracted the lymph node, then a biopsy was performed on it. Later, Beth and I met with the doctor, who gave us the news. This ball-like mass was a collection of plasma cells that had found their way into the lymph system—collecting in the gland under my left arm. They call this a "plasmacytoma." He said, "This is considered cancer because these plasma cells do not belong there. Anytime cells are located where they usually don't occur, it's considered cancerous." He added that during the operation, they found no other noticeable irregularities. I understood that the cells were just in the wrong spot. But my wife, and mother of our two sons, heard "Cancer!" We made an appointment for me to meet with an oncologist.

On short notice, Dr. Brennan, an oncologist, met with us. He examined me and interviewed me about my health. He was not convinced of the conclusion arrived at in the pathology report, because it was not the norm for a man my age, 40 years old and in excellent health, to have an occurrence of such cancer. Additionally, it was odd that there were no other symptoms, such as pain or fatigue, that often accompany it.

This type of cancer is primarily located in the bones and, usually later, it is metastasized into soft tissue, and I did not have any of the symptoms of this type of cancer. He indicated that he wanted to see the pathology samples himself. He would wait until after seeing them before sending me for any further testing or recommending a course of action.

We left his office with me feeling very optimistic about the possibility that everything was being blown out of proportion. I felt optimistic. Besides, in a few days, we would be leaving the cold of a Kentucky winter to visit my in-laws in Melbourne, Florida, for a week (my father-in-law has since passed away), expecting it to be a relaxing experience.

Our drive to Melbourne, Florida, to see Grandma Mo and Papa Donut, with the two boys, went well. Early in the week, I played golf with my father-in-law. Well, he played a round while I took a golf course tour, looking for my ball. We went to the beach and to Cape Canaveral to watch a shuttle launch, which was postponed. Then, midweek, I flew home to see Dr. Brennan and hear some good news, or maybe not.

As he entered the room, I thought, "Well, doc, tell me what I already know. This is a mistake, and I have nothing to worry about." Dr. Brennan has a matter-of-fact kind of demeanor when you talk with him, as you might expect; the personalities of pilots as a whole are a "just the facts" type group. I am tuned into this approach.

He began by telling me he had seldom seen anyone my age with good health practices with a plasmacytoma and no other symptoms. He looked at my pathology samples, and there was no doubt that it was a plasmacytoma. His concern became, was there anything else of more significant concern going on in my body that hadn't yet revealed itself and was not determined by this biopsy? A plasmacytoma rarely occurs by itself.

He was ordering blood draws, full-body X-rays, a CAT scan, MRI, and various other tests. "I'll be in touch to let you know when. Do you have any questions?" "Ahh...." I had one of those blindsided moments that often arise from the unexpected and when you are not knowledgeable enough to know what questions to ask. "No," was my reply.

I headed home to call Beth in Florida to give her the news and leave her to contemplate what this may mean for her and our family. Alone that night in our new house, gave me plenty of time to think about what the doctor had said. Oddly enough, my lack of understanding of the seriousness of everything the doctor told me gave me the opportunity for a good night's sleep.

The next day, I flew back to my family with a different view of what was important in my life. That became apparent to me when we took our son Noah to Cape Canaveral, who was just two years old and interested in rockets—not to go on a tour but to just show him the rockets close up. However, they were behind a fence, and it cost 24 dollars for each person to go through the gate to see the rocket display.

Usually, I would have thought, "Twenty-four dollars just to walk around some rockets; I don't think so." But life had just taken a turn down an unknown road. Beth thought I was crazy when frugal me paid for each of us, so that Noah could run and climb around the rocket display. That little boy had no idea what his daddy was about to face, nor did I. He was in the moment, and it was time to join him. My job took me away from my family too much, and I wanted positive memories for the unknown journey ahead.

Chapter 2

Reality Happens

"Reality is merely an illusion, albeit a very persistent one."
– Albert Einstein

After our return from Florida, I spent a few days taking care of all the tests the doctor had determined were necessary. Once he had the results, he could choose a prognosis and what course of action to take.

When the test results came back, it was good news. It appeared that I had a single, solitary plasmacytoma. The full body X-rays showed no active spots or lesions on my skeletal structure, nor were there any other spots in my soft tissues or organs. Yeah! The only caveat was that my blood contained a protein. It was not cut and dry as to the significance of that blood protein level for me personally. While it is not customary to have that particular protein in your blood, knowing the level before removing the plasmacytoma would have been helpful with the prognosis.

The plan was for me to receive radiation treatments to destroy any undetected remaining malignant cells. The radiation therapy introduced me to doctor Dr. John Sacco; his specialty is radiation oncology. He laid out the plan and explained centralized radiation's purpose of the treatments concentrated on my left underarm area. The regimen would be five days a week for five weeks, and I should expect some burning on the skin, similar to a harsh sunburn. He recommended that I apply aloe vera gel to the area twice daily, along with vitamin E oil, to help with the discomfort and healing.

But before it began, I had to talk to my boss, the chief pilot, about my predicament and why I wanted an extended leave of absence from work. The secretary was familiar with pilots who, in the past, required some time off to deal with cancers, and told me that I could expect a minimum of six months off. I gave her the starting date of my treatments and then went off to fly my trip.

I don't recall his name, but I remember the first officer being funny and energetic. He had me laughing and entertained by his commentary during the four days we flew together. Flight deck crews work as a team, whether they fly for airlines, corporations, or in the military. A tremendous amount of money is spent training them, with safety as a top priority. A part of that "safety first" approach to everything we do, is learning about human factors. We call it crew resource management, or CRM. It includes listening and observing your partner to notice subtle irregularities in their standard operating procedures, communications, or inconsistencies.

During the last flight of the four days, I was quiet and did not respond much to my first officer's repertoire of humor. It had hit home with me that maybe this was the end of my flying career. It was a journey that started when I was sixteen, and I took my first lesson with the money I earned by flipping hamburgers. It was a childhood dream realized through sacrifice, focus, patience, and failures along the way. What if the FAA did not let me return to flying?

Pulling into the gate, I remarked that this might be my last time in the cockpit. The first officer said, "Whoa, what's up?" I gave him a cliff note version of what had been going on in my life for the last few months. He remarked that he had thought something was bothering me. Then he quipped, "I thought it was serious like your wife left you and took your dog and pick-up truck," minor jovial harassment about me being from Kentucky. I laughed. "Why didn't you say something?" he added. "Man, you should've flown that leg."

I said goodbye to the cabin crew and walked up the jet bridge into a rarely vacant terminal in Charlotte, North Carolina. There I ran into a favorite captain of mine, Jim Black, (now retired and passed on) whom I had flown with as his first officer. He and I had become friends and had gone to many places across the globe scuba diving together, along with other friends I met through him. He asked, "How's it going?" I said, "Jim, I may have just flown my last flight." He wanted an explanation. I shared with him what was going on. His response was, "Cancer, you?" Yep, me.

During my visits with Dr. John Sacco, I learned of his interest in the integrative approach to medicine. We talked many times about numerous things, including what he has learned about foods and other natural ways to combat cancer. Through our discussions, he realized that healthy living was something I was doing before my diagnosis. On one of my visits, he presented me with a few pages of references of scientific reports on alternative and Integrative therapies, which he had gotten from attending oncology symposiums.

After the five weeks of radiation, I said my farewells to the staff at the cancer center and some patients I had met, wishing them a successful journey. Also, a brief conversation with Doctor Sacco ended with his courteous, "If there is ever anything I can do for you, call me." Little did we know that our paths would cross again.

Chapter 3

Mirror, Mirror on the Wall

"Reality continues to ruin my life."
– Bill Watterson, *The Complete Calvin and Hobbes*

September 11, 2001, shook the United States to its core, like the attack on Pearl Harbor in 1941 when it propelled us into the Second World War. This act of terrorism also started the airline industry down a road of accelerated change. By 2004, my company had filed for Chapter 11 bankruptcy. With the reorganization, the airline shrunk to half its size. My personal compensation was greatly reduced, along with the loss of my pension. But I was one of the lucky ones. I still had my job. Many of my colleagues were on the street, jobless.

Things were not going so well with work. My flight schedule increased, and our finances were in a predicament. We added our new son, Joseph. Life for my wife Beth was much busier and more challenging. Additionally, my days away increased to about 22 each month. How this new normal affected my family became apparent when I corrected my oldest son, Noah, at the dinner table one evening. He responded, "You're not the boss; mom's the boss, and you're never home!" I was speechless and emotionally stabbed in the heart by a six-year-old boy speaking from his soul. He was right. Stress was in ample supply in our home. But in proper natural form, Beth adjusted and did a fantastic job keeping our home and family organized and a happy environment to come home to.

Around this time, I began to notice the skin around my belt line was changing color. It started as one quarter size spot on one hip, then one on the other. Strange, yes, but I thought little of it. As months went by, the two areas grew and began to migrate around my hips, leaving wrinkled skin behind.

Over a period of about four years, the discoloration continued to expand along my waist and began to migrate to my buttocks. But it was not until the jowls on my face appeared that my ego started to get the best of me. I heeded Beth's recommendation to see a dermatologist. I pick a top dermatologist in the area and made an appointment.

The discoloring from my hip area continued to grow during the time before the appointment. It was moving down to my posterior and up to my abdomen. Each morning when I woke, the first thing I would see in the mirror was my aging face staring back at me. Additionally, I had developed a "turkey neck" appearance. I had gone from being a "kid-looking" pilot, of whom some passengers wondered if I was old enough to drive a car, to being asked by my fellow pilots how many years I had left before retirement. I was only 44 years of age.

Finally, the day came. After he had looked me over, he decided a biopsy was necessary.

I returned the following week and had a biopsy in his office, and it was sent to a lab. The report identified my skin as Cutis Laxa, a condition of the connective tissue, reducing the elastin in the dermal layers and causing a loosening of the skin, much like when we age.

Okay, doc, now what do we do about it? He gave me a prescription for an ointment to apply to my skin. I followed the doctor's recommended regimen while continuing to see him. I asked several times about the loose skin on my neck and face. I received an answer similar to, "Well, when you lose a lot of weight, your skin can loosen because of being previously stretched.' Hmm, I weighed the same as when I graduated from high school more than 25 years ago.

That's it. Next! I began my search for a new dermatologist.

I had quarterly appointments with Dr. Brennan, my oncologist. He would do a series of blood tests and thoroughly inspect my physical self. The blood protein of unknown origin was stable, and that was good. During these visits, he asked me how I was feeling. I answered, "Great! I am still running and working out." In passing, I did mention my skin condition. He looked at the area in question but did not offer any suggestions. After all, he was an oncologist. It had nothing to do with my plasmacytoma in the past. Well, that was good.

I began researching Cutis Laxa. I discovered it was a condition that was only found in as few as 300 hundred families worldwide, according to a University of Pittsburgh web page. It is usually inherited. But in sporadic cases, older adults acquire it due to another condition, including being tied to a blood protein of unknown origin. "BIngo."

Checking with many dermatologists for an appointment, I learned the shortest available time was six months. Visiting with my mom one day and explaining my plight to her, my sister Judy, a nurse, walked in and heard my saga about finding a timely appointment. She asked me what type of doctor I was interested in seeing. I wanted a female dermatologist who was relatively new. Why, you ask? First, women are typically better at listening and more empathetic than men. Secondly, I believed that if she was still fresh to the field, she might be more open-minded and up on the newest possibilities for treatment. She made a phone call, and I had an appointment with Dr. Stephanie Snyder within two weeks.

During the first meeting with her, she listened. She examined my skin and had some ideas about what it could be. But she said she would like to do a biopsy. Been there, done that. I agreed and asked, "When?" "Now, if you have the time?" was her response. "This is wonderful," I thought. "This lady will not delay trying to figure this out and recognizes my time is just as valuable as hers. No reason to schedule it for another day." A big "Yeah!" for her.

She told me to drop my drawers so that she could stick some needles into my posterior, aka my butt cheeks. "Doc, we just met," I joked. Now, that is not the ideal spot for someone who sits on the job all day. I questioned her choice. She answered, "It is the least painful because of the fatty tissue. Just like when you were a little kid and received shots from the doctor."

"Okay then, take some samples of my buttocks for science and research," I thought. I jumped up on the table in my underwear. It was one of those times when I heard my mother's voice, "I hope you had a decent pair of underwear on." She stuck me in the rear. Then she sewed up the hole (not that one) and made an appointment to review the results. Out the door, I went.

When I met with Dr. Snyder to discuss the biopsy results, she told me it appeared I have a condition called Cutsis Laxa. Okay, we had an agreement with the other doctor. The question was, "Why do you have it at this point in your life since it is commonly a hereditary condition that appears in a young child?" She admittedly could not answer that question.

She invited her partner in, and we had a meeting of our minds of possible next steps. One included me going to a conference of dermatologists to expose my wrinkles. Finally, we agreed on trying to schedule an appointment with Dr. Callen, who at that time was the head of the department of dermatology at the University of Louisville medical school.

Doctor Callen reviewed the information sent to him by Dr. Snyder, and he agreed to see me. On the day of my appointment, I drove two hours to Louisville, Kentucky, to meet with him. When we met, he told me to loosen my clothing. I stood there while he and some medical students looked me over. He agreed with Dr. Snyder's diagnosis. Then he added, "The question is, what is going on to trigger it at this point in your life?" He elected to take some blood samples. Oh, how I have come to love those needles. I also agreed to let him take photos of my bare body to share with his colleagues and the world of dermatology. I stripped down to pose for my "glamour shots." It was embarrassingly chilly that day.

Within a few weeks, I received a letter from Dr. Callen, and my oncologist also received one. In the letter was the acknowledgment of the protein in my blood, called monoclonal gammopathy protein, of unknown origin, of which Dr. Brennan was aware. It was not long before I heard from Dr. Brennan and of his plan to run me through a whole battery of tests like I had done eight years earlier. Again, they took a quart of my blood. Well, it seemed like a quart with all the vials they filled. Then there were full body X-rays, an MRI, and all the other tests they did the first time.

When the results came back, the diagnosis was active multiple myeloma. For the unfamiliar, myeloma is a plasma or white blood cell cancer. Healthy plasma cells typically generate antibodies, which the immune system uses to attack foreign pathogens. Abnormal white blood cells produce irregular antibodies. Myeloma comes to us from the Greek word for marrow, "myelo," and "oma," meaning tumor. These plasma cells form an accumulation of irregular cells in the bones, weakening them by replacing normal plasma cells with myeloma cells, leading to many breaks in one's bones and the loss of density of the bones. As a result of loss of bone density, a person with multiple myeloma can also experience a loss of height. I met several men and a woman who had lost two and as much as eight inches because of the disease. The "multiple" title comes from being active in many areas. In my case, it was the skull, ribs, spine, and hips.

Stunned, I asked myself, "What now?"

Chapter 4

Experience Shapes Our Truth

"Facts do not cease to exist because they are ignored."
– Aldous Huxley

To lay the foundation for my determination to win, please indulge me as I tell a story of my youth, because I believe it is essential to know the mindset needed to meet life's challenges.

When I was seventeen, I made a thoughtless choice; I dove into shallow water and broke my neck. As I lay in the water, I heard "the voice," the same one that had told me not to dive in, but I did not listen. This time I did, and it said, "Get your head out of the water before you drown." I stood up and collapsed back into a sitting position in shallower water that came to my waistline. I thought I would be okay, thinking I had just taken a blow to the head and got a "stinger," a tingling sensation all over my body, now known to be a symptom of a concussion.

Soon I realized I was not okay. As I began to see clearly, I noticed that the water running down my face had a red tint as it passed in front of my eyes. "Oh, oh, something's wrong with this picture," I thought. I am forever grateful to a nurse, who happened to be there. Or was she there as part of a more fantastic plan? She assisted me and possibly saved me from being a quadriplegic, or even my life, according to the doctors who later evaluated me at Cincinnati Children's Hospital. She did a quick evaluation on the riverbank and realized I could not move my limbs normally on my left side. Movement of my arms and legs was minimal and time limited, but there was some feeling in my fingers.

People there helped to move me out of the water to the riverbank while my new nurse friend immobilized my head and neck to prevent further damage to my spine. I am forever grateful, mystery nurse. One of her companions drove to find a phone (before cell phones) to call an ambulance. The emergency personnel came through a cornfield to load me into my ride to the emergency room. After an evaluation at a small hospital in Indiana, transportation was arranged to Cincinnati's Children's Hospital in Cincinnati, Ohio. There I was operated on to immobilize my neck and put me in traction for an undetermined amount of time—a glorious way to celebrate my graduation from high school and spend summer vacation.

As I lay there with no place to go, my parents brought me some recordings of the late but excellent motivator, Zig Ziglar. They hoped I would listen. Well, what else could I do? I was flat on my back in traction. When no one was visiting, I would listen. Hearing his words nurtured my already present positive determination, and I developed a sense of "How can I ...?"

This contributed to my determination to walk again. Within one month, I went from lying flat on my back in traction from a vertebrae injury that, if it had slid any further, would have ended my life, to roaming the hallways of the hospital. Why wouldn't I choose positive thinking as a lifestyle? I do give credit for my favorable outcome to having a top doctor for neurological injuries, at the **University of Cincinnati Medical Center**, the late Dr. McLuren.

Governing our universe are many natural laws. One of these laws is the law of cause and effect, stated simply as, "Every action has a reaction or consequence." Or as the Bible says, "What we sow, so also shall we reap." This applies to the choices we make. Our choices, or lack of, affects our outcomes. Decisions to act may be a result of fear-filled helplessness or can be action oriented to face a challenge. Your choices are either self-empowering or self-defeating and will influence the outcome of the circumstances at hand. Our perception of the situation will influence what we choose to do. Is it one of the positive possibilities or of victimhood? If you believe you have some influence over the situation, you will take steps towards the outcome you want. If you feel hopeless, then your belief is, "Why bother?"

Back to the cancer journey. So, being Mister Positive, I was not phased by the oncologist's news, right? Nope. In fact, all I heard was, "You are going to die!" Well, that is not what he said, but that is the meaning my mind put to the explanation of a three-to-seven-year life span for people who have multiple myeloma.

Now it was time to go home and break the news to my lovely bride. When we sat down to talk, I explained to her the best I could, with my lack of understanding of the disease, what we were about to face as a family. My ignorance at the time of my situation enabled me to keep a positive spin on our conversation. In my heart, I believe in many ways the journey for her has been more difficult, stressful, and emotionally draining than for me. After all, I could focus on the battle at hand. She was looking beyond the moment, to her life as a single parent.

After much discussion over many days, Beth and I elected to tell our boys. One night after dinner, we called the boys back to the dinner table. When eight-year-old Noah heard the word cancer, he cried. I am unsure of what he understood about it. But he did know it was not good news. He was familiar with people at his school who had lost loved ones to the disease. When I saw the tears in his eyes, I cried for the first time. I had spent a lot of time worrying about what was going to happen to my family, and what would the result be of my boys not growing up with their father, or how their mother would be able to provide for them.

My curious first grader, Chris, asked me some very good questions. The one I remember best was, "Can I catch this disease from you?" I assured him he could not. I thought, "God bless you little man." I wanted to let him know that even though Dad had tears in his eyes, it was going to be okay. But at the time, I did not believe it myself. It really brought home the fact that my career as an airline pilot had taken me away from them far too much.

Joseph, our funny guy, was too young at three to get it. When I mentioned that I wanted to laugh a lot, he took up the request as a mission to put a smile on my face. He has many silly facial expressions, leading one of his uncles to label him as "Joe Carey," after the comedic actor Jim Carey and his notable expressions. He has a comical way of looking at life, which when I think about his take on things, makes me laugh. If only, as adults, we could find the humor he does through observing life, and then pausing and seeing just how weird it can be.

He is not one to say, "When we look back on this, we'll laugh." No, he laughs now. What a gift that is and one I wish I had. I think he got it from his mother, who is also gleeful.

As I mentioned, the most difficult part for me was how this was going to affect my family. Yet, that also became one of the most motivating questions I asked myself. My answer was to choose life. To me, that meant that my focus was going to be finding what I could do to make the time I had with my family more of joy and less of worry, as well as doing my part to extend my physical existence and, at the very least, to feel as good as possible during the journey. But most importantly, I was going to focus on being as emotionally positive as I could make myself, so that emotionally, I would not bring the whole family along for the ride—they did not deserve it.

My mom taught me, while I was lying flat on my back in the hospital, in traction with a broken neck, not to ask "why me" questions. Put the "why" in the past. Instead, "What am I going to do about it?" or "How can I change or use this to move forward?" are far more effective questions to ask yourself when creating a better future than the one that seems to be apparent in the present. Reflecting on what my mother taught me, what was I going to do about this cancer? How could I change and move forward? Though I felt like I was doing all the right things to live a long and healthy life, there was room for improvement.

It was investigation time.

Chapter 5
Curiosity Wins Over Fear

Many want 1000s of things.
The sick want only one... health.
– Undetermined

The beauty of the internet is that there is a wealth of information accessible to people, with little difficulty and little effort. The scariest thing about the internet is that there is a wealth of information accessible to people, with little difficulty and little effort. No, that is not a misprint. Information can be valuable, or it can be misleading. Anyone can post or say anything on the internet unchallenged, without considering its accuracy or validity. I am not saying that the information on the internet is worthless. It's just a reminder of the importance of authenticating sources of what you read and hear.

To ensure you are finding accurate information, follow the three D's:

Dates. Check when the information was first available and for updates on the subject. Just because it's not dated does not mean it is recent. There may be updated information on the topic.

Documentation. Verify the sources. Are they from respected science journals? The Health on the Net (HON) Foundation seal indicates reliable and credible material.

Double-check. It is okay and suggested to be skeptical. Comparing information from several sources to find supporting research increases validation. Double-checking with your doctor before following any advice from the net is prudent.

One of the first areas was to try and understand just what cancer is. An understandable explanation came from Gary Null, Ph.D., in his book *Overcoming Cancer*. Tissue is a group of cells combined to make up the organs and bones of the body. Every cell has a blueprint of genetic information the body uses for growth and repair. As cells develop and mature, an internal maintenance mechanism enables them to repair themselves when possible. However, if the cell does not evolve properly, or has reached its effectiveness, this mechanism programs it to die. Cancer occurs when this process of growth, repair, maturity, and then programmed death does not materialize and starts to replicate. In layperson's terms, cancer is a group of cells that don't play by the rules.

When choosing a doctor, it is valuable to determine if they are aware of and open to including holistic possibilities. I recalled the conversations with my radiation oncologist, Doctor John Sacco, about the treatments for plasmacytoma. He had spoken of the importance of incorporating personal lifestyle changes when facing a cancer diagnosis. Reconnecting with him, I asked if he had any suggestions I could incorporate into the treatment plans. He recommended that I read a book written by Doctor Keith Block, titled *Life Over Cancer*; adding at the time, Doctor Block was one of the more popular speakers at oncologist conventions. I got a copy of his book and started reading.

After completing his book, I included him in my medical mastermind of valuable assets in my crusade against this chronic cancer disease. In my conversation with Doctor Keith Block at the **Block Center's Integrative Cancer Treatment Center** in Chicago, Illinois, he told me that my options were not limited to conventional practices. This comprehensive approach to integrative therapy is what his program is centered around: creating a plan that encompasses chemotherapy along with lifestyle changes, a more plant-centric diet, an assessment of the environment in which I live my life, and possible therapies found outside typical Western medicine.

With research going on all the time, everything is in a constant state of change. About every three to five years, something new comes into the oncology field. Each year you can continue your cancer battle may lend itself to another possibility of the latest discoveries becoming available. Be open to new possibilities, but identify the source as valid and reliable, not just "they said."

I encourage you to investigate nutrition and how foods can benefit or hinder all aspects of your health. I am sure you will find plenty of information to digest. (Was that a pun?) Your research will help lead you to your own conclusions. Let this be your warning that many in the medical community firmly believe it is not worthy of consideration if it does not come from a laboratory-produced liquid or pill. And I am not advocating ignoring conventional therapies. Please let the doctors do what they do, and you take care of the things in your control.

Chemotherapy treatments hammer the body with toxins, intending to kill the cancerous cells. Still, these chemicals also slay the healthy ones. Your body needs food to rebuild the good cells necessary for your survival. Consuming foods known to be beneficial enables the body to function and rebuild naturally, which can affect how you will feel during the therapy.

The first step to being a victor is to take control of the things you can manage, like your diet. The adage from the computer world of "garbage in, garbage out" also applies to the body. This internal ecosystem needs balance to serve you in an intended way. One of the best things you can do to contribute to this balance is to make every effort to supply it adequately with valuable nutrients.

I elected to emphasize the quality of calories over quantity and cajoled myself into eating even when I did not want to, ensuring that the foods were nutritionally beneficial. Admittedly, I indulged, and still do, in yummy desserts occasionally. If it includes dark chocolate, I ate it and still do. But, hey, research supports dark chocolate as being medicinal. That's my excuse.

The closer you get to nature's food, the more valuable the chemical compositions naturally present to provide the body nutritionally. Science refers to these as phytochemicals or phytonutrients. Phyto comes from the Greek word for plant. These valuable chemicals have names such as isoflavonoids, carotenoids, and stilbenoids, of which resveratrol, found in red wine, may be the most commonly known. There are more than 25,000 other possible known naturally occurring substances. Each of them protects the plant from threats from its environment, such as germs, pests, diseases, and others that affect the plant. Many pharmaceuticals come from these chemicals found in plants.

My choice is to turn my focus to eating more, not exclusively, plant food of wide varieties, as I have heard it referred to as living food versus dead food. A diet rich in plants contains more nutritionally adequate disease-fighting compounds than an animal protein-centric diet. Eating as close to the food's original state as possible provides:

- More minerals and healthy blends for the body.
- The ability to put them to work.
- Protection from daily exposure to toxins in our homes, work, and overall environment.

If consuming meat or fish, consider that animals fed an organic diet, including healthy grains and grasses, pass the benefits of those foods on to the people who consume them as part of their diet. For example, chickens that eat grains abundant in omega-3 fatty acids, have eggs more plentiful in those compounds than those not raised with a diet plentiful in omega-3s. Likewise, when a person drinks the milk or eats the meat of livestock given hormones and antibiotics, these concoctions are transferred to the one consuming them. If you like animal protein, consider focusing on quality raised stock, such as grass-fed beef and free-range chickens. Yes, they are higher in cost, but they have lower chemical exposure, improved quality, and are better for you.

Chapter 6

S.A.D.

"If diet is wrong, medicine is of no use."
– Ancient Ayurvedic Proverb

If you live in the United States, food is abundantly available in grocery stores and our many restaurants. The problem is that we, as a population, have developed poor eating habits. SAD, the Standard American Diet, is precisely that, sad. With incredible consumption of low-nutrient value foods and high trans fats, we have an epidemic of chronic diseases in a land of astonishing abundance.

The U.S. experiences higher rates of cancer and a decreased life span when compared to some other countries; for example, Japan. One of the most recognizable dietary differences between Japan and the United States may be more extensive exposure to convenience foods, and fast-food restaurants. The Japanese, who consume fewer refined sugars, less land animal proteins, and lower bad fats, fare better. Though they still have incidents of cancer, it progresses more slowly or becomes less advanced, both in women and men, thereby living longer.

The American diet tends to be greater in simple carbohydrates and higher in damaging fats, leading to larger body fat ratios with increased weight. The trans-fats associated with partially hydrogenated oils—think snack foods—tend to be promoters of ill health. In addition, a poor diet weakens the immune system and increases oxidative stress in the body, multiplying internal inflammation. These promote tumor growth and possible mutations in the DNA, supporting more aggressive cancers and making them more challenging to beat.

Chronic inflammation often goes undetected until it culminates in conditions such as arthritis, heart disease, diabetes, and cancer. This chronic condition overproduces inflammatory agents, disrupting the biological balance, and neutralizing a part of the immune system. Some factors known to increase the risk of chronic inflammation are smoking, stress, sleep problems, and a diet high in trans fats. Metastasis, or the growth and spread of cancer cells, relies on pro-inflammatory agents to block the immune system's standard biological response to mutated cells, enabling an irregular cell continuous life and not subjecting them to the natural reaction of cell death that the body would do when the system operates appropriately.

Part of the body's response to healing is angiogenesis when new blood vessels grow in areas needing mending. Unfortunately, it can be "hijacked" by malignant growths, helping cancer cells thrive. High glycemic foods, such as white flour-based products, release insulin and insulin growth factor (IGF), stimulating a surge of cancer cells. In addition, high glycemic foods facilitate inflammation, acting as a "fertilizer" to tumor cells. Now we have a double whammy; not only is this sweetened blood environment favorable to cancer growth, but insulin can add fuel to the fire of several cancers, including the colon and breast.

The **Journal of Clinical Oncology** reported that women with the highest blood insulin levels were twice as likely to experience a reappearance of breast cancer after remission. Also, it was more likely to spread to other parts of the body, by up to 300 percent, compared to women with lower glucose levels. The excellent news is that preliminary findings in lab experiments indicate that lowering blood sugar levels in animals leads to higher survival rates. It is important to note that avoiding high glycemic foods associated with a simple carbohydrate-rich diet is necessary.

A **European Journal of Cancer** study, investigating cancer and nutrition, involved more than 500,000 people living in 10 different nations. The analysis revealed a positive relationship between reduced incidents of cancers among those who ate foods high in phytonutrients and foods rich in antioxidants. These nutrients are often associated with a Mediterranean diet, with its high intake of fruits, vegetables, fish, fiber, and calcium-abundant ones such as yogurt or kefir. Studies indicate that a healthy lifestyle and a quality diet are associated with reduced inflammation. Changing harmful habits and avoiding low-value foods promotes better health, improving our chances of cancer-free living.

A nutritional therapy program is a component of an integrative approach to increase your prospects of success. To create an anti-cancer diet, the emphasis must be on plant foods and significantly avoiding refined meats. Published in **Lancet Oncology**, evidence accumulated by hundreds of studies, and reviewed by hundreds of experts, established that eating as little as 50 grams of processed meat, the equivalent of one hot dog or four strips of bacon a day, can increase the prospects of colorectal cancer. But don't panic, because the **International Agency for Research on Cancer** has classified the quantity of these foods as the culprit, so an occasional BLT or sausage with your morning breakfast is tolerable.

The consumption of healthy nourishment affects blood chemistry and strengthens the body's ability to respond to all disorders. Evidence supports the concept that foods are valuable to both defeating as well as stopping the development of cancer at the outset. The **American Cancer Society** advocates restricting unhealthy, simple carbohydrates and high-fat meats. A high-fat diet can impair anti-cancer mechanisms such as natural killer (NK) cells. At the same time, an increase in NK cell activity and a low-fat diet are related.

Chapter 7

Food Is Thy Medicine

"Health is about the life you gain."
– Dr. Josh Axe

If a poor diet can have negative consequences, why couldn't a nutrient-rich one have positive effects on health?

The intake of nutrient-rich foods can adjust the body's biology, helping to indirectly control the spread of cancer by providing valuable vitamins and minerals needed to discourage cancer cell progression. To match the spirit-draining effects of chemotherapy and radiation treatments, you need life-giving energy. Having the stamina to meet the up and down cycles that come from these therapies empowers you to actively engage in the process of fighting the disease while rebuilding yourself physically as well as mentally. Emphasize high-fiber carbohydrates, including fresh fruits and veggies. Good plant protein sources are available from lentils, beans, peas, and other legumes. Following the recommendations of the **American Medical Association** of limiting high-fat meats, slashing refined sugar intake, and consuming fewer starches like bread, rice, and white potatoes, along with getting regular exercise, can cut mortality rates.

Your victor's diet prioritizes plant foods since they provide valuable phytochemicals and micronutrients. These healthy foods are essential to reducing the internal inflammation, lowering the risk of cancer and tumor growth and progression. Avoiding animal products is important because many receive hormone treatments, antibiotics, and toxins in their feed. In some studies, there are indications of higher rates of cell DNA mutations when exposed particularly to red meat.

The following discussion is about some foods known to have cancer fighting compounds put there by nature, that may contribute to interrupting the metastatic process. This is not to be an exhaustive discussion of all the possibilities, since that is beyond the scope of this book. Its purpose is to inform the reader about what worked for me, and to get you started in your own investigations.

When I received my second cancer diagnosis, I knew it was time to make some changes. One area that I could improve upon quickly and has been identified as influencing cancer development in the body is diet. Studies propose a simple lifestyle change, like a healthier diet, can prevent a large percentage of cancers. According to the **American Institute for Cancer Research**, 47 percent of colon cancers are preventable through diet and lifestyle changes.

A buzzword commonly recited in the alternative health world is "superfoods." What makes a food "super?" There is not necessarily any scientific basis for this classification. The term is generally assigned to foods that are high in valuable nutrients and are considered to contain health and healing properties. It is largely more of a marketing term. They don't have to be exotic or crazy expensive to make the list. You could grow them in your backyard or buy them at a farmer's market or most any food stores that stock fresh produce.

Plants have an abundance of phytonutrients or organic chemicals generated by the plant to protect it and help it flourish in its environment. Many of these natural compounds, researchers have found, support cellular health and may have curative properties. For instance, in laboratory mice, sulforaphane, a phytochemical abundant in cruciferous vegetables like broccoli and cauliflower, was identified in studies as a substance shown to reduce tumors.

Normal bodily functions generate oxidative stressors called free radicals, that disrupt the biological balance and the body's natural defenses. Accelerated aging and increased risk of diabetes and cancer have been linked to this imbalance. The natural variety of antioxidants contained in a plant-based diet, offers oxidative protection by offsetting free radicals and helping to regulate a person's biological operations.

To start the discussion, we will look at the more potent foods in battling cancer. There are many vegetables available to us to include in our daily diets. Learning to integrate wholesome foods into your day is possible with some effort and planning. Eating them will also improve many areas of overall health. These culinary superstars positively affect physical and mental wellness, including diabetes, cardiovascular, neurological, psychological, and even emotional well-being. Almost anything related to healthy well-being and longevity is influenced by these foods.

Tea Time

One of my first adjustments was to begin to drink green tea regularly. This is significant for me when compared to the commercially produced fruit juices I was often consuming. Those are high in sugar and calories and are limited in nutritional value, and as noted, cancer loves sugar.

Green tea contains small molecular compounds called catechins. Clinical studies have established a positive correlation between these polyphenolic compounds and controlling oxidative stress, anti-inflammatory, and anti-proliferation of cancer cells within the body, by blocking unregulated growth of blood vessels needed to promote the spread of cancer. One of the most examined and powerful of these catechins is epigallocatechin gallate, or EGCG. EGCG catechins act as chemo-preventative or chemotherapeutic agents in various types of cancers, and it may be an effective booster of some drugs used to treat them. The **Mayo Clinic** has listed it as having significant clinical benefits for leukemia and lymph node-related cancers. They recommend drinking large quantities of green tea daily. In laboratory studies, these catechin flavonoids are attributed to having significant effects on human health. The catechins EGC and EGCG in green tea appear to be very potent, being as much as 100 percent more effective than the antioxidants vitamin C and E.

Research with mice orally given green tea polyphenols (GTP), documented a reduction in skin cancer incidence from UVB rays, lower numbers of malignancies per animal, and a slower rate of tumor growth. Relative to prostate cancer (PCA), the most common form of non-skin cancer for American men, GTP created a meaningful suspension of additional cancer development, and a significant reduction in the size of existing tumors, while restraining the progression of new cancer cells to distant organ sites. The dosage was the equivalent of six cups of green tea each day.

Breast cancer cells' tendency to easily invade other tissues in the body is a reason for the high mortality rate of breast cancer patients. Research notes a positive correlation between the consumption of more than five cups a day of green tea, with a reduction in stage I and II breast cancer. **Clinical Cancer Research**, a peer reviewed medical journal on oncology, reported that while examining the effects of GTP on the growth and spread of mouse mammary carcinoma in a laboratory, scientists also noted an induction of apoptosis, increasing the survival rates.

In tests introducing green tea catechins in laboratory mice, there was an advancement in the activity of natural killer cells, when compared to mice that did not receive EGCG. **Experimental Lung Research**, a peer-reviewed medical journal that publishes articles in the respiratory field, reported that a nutrient rich mix of vitamin C, the amino acids lysine, the protein creating proline, arginine, and green tea extract, was given to laboratory mice. After two weeks of receiving this mixture, the mice had a 63% reduction in lung cancer growth.

Liver cancer is increasing all over the world, with limited effective treatments available. The same nutrient mixture of vitamin C, lysine, proline, arginine, and green tea extract was given to some laboratory mice that had liver cancer cells, while others received a regular diet. Highlighted in **Oncology Reports**, the supplemental group experienced a reduction in the growth and spread of the malignant cells, and an increase in survival.

There were other promising responses recorded about the inclusion of GTP as a part of a personal chemotherapeutic effort. Richard Béliveau, currently the director of the **Molecular Medicine Laboratory** and a researcher in the **Department of Neurosurgery at Notre-Dame Hospital** in Montreal, Canada, lists EGCG from green tea in his book, *Foods That Fight Cancer*. It acts as a powerful blocking agent against the growth of new cancer cells by hindering the development of new blood vessels. It also establishes itself on the surfaces of new cells, creating a barrier to the receptors that grant cancer cells access to surrounding tissue. Furthermore, green tea acts as a detoxifier for the body.

The interest in GTP as a personal therapeutic is being studied extensively, and evidence documenting EGC and EGCG's effects against the spread of cancers is growing. Since the majority of cancer deaths are related to the metastasis of the primary tumor to other areas in the body, preventing its spread would be impactful. The inclusion of innovative therapeutic agents like those found in green tea, along with more early detection strategies for cancer, could be valuable to successful outcomes.

Green Envy

To live well and promote good health, it is a must to have a diet rich in vitamins and minerals. Leafy greens are essential to a foundation of strength and well-being. In addition to their crucial vitamins and minerals, they also provide valuable antioxidants, along with enzymes needed to properly digest and absorb nutrients and breakdown blood toxins, and other functions.

An array of various leafy greens offers significant intrinsic nutrients; spinach and arugula were the ones that I ate most often. There is considerable research available on the cancer fighting abilities of these vegetables, while also contributing antibacterial and antiviral properties. Additionally, they are a source of glucosinolates. During digestion, it breaks down into a powerful sulfur compound called isothiocyanates, known for their anticarcinogenic activity as well as interfering with metastasis.

According to the **International Journal of Vitamin and Nutritional Research**, this effect was studied both in a Petri dish as well as in human tissue experiments. Isothiocyanates were observed inhibiting the duplication of malignant cells, and induced apoptosis in human cancer cells, along with the strong anti-inflammatory and antioxidant attributes, protecting cells from damage. Glucosinolates can be an incredibly weapon in a personal battle to win over cancer.

One of the leafy greens I consume in large amounts is spinach. It is an excellent source of the essential mineral iron, and important for the development of hemoglobin, which is what carries oxygen in the blood to the body's organs and tissues. Spinach also contains the supportive vitamins and minerals of calcium, magnesium, and potassium, and vitamins A, C, B6, E, and folic acid, all crucial to the healthy functioning of the muscles, heart, and nervous system. All are essential to maintaining normal body operations.

Spinach leaves have a rich concentration of carotenoids. These antioxidants enhance the immune system as well as disease protection. A diet that includes foods with high levels of antioxidants can strengthen the ability of the body to fight cancers and provide protective benefits to healthy cells.

In numerous studies conducted on the potential of a plant-based diet offering a reduction in cancer risks, spinach is one of those plants having a plentiful array of naturally occurring nutrient bullets that help to decrease the possibility of cancer. One of the powerful carotenoids in spinach is a group called glycolipids. In laboratory experiments, these compounds were found to inhibit the ability of cervix cancer cells to duplicate themselves.

Yes, these carotenoids were in a controlled environment. However, what if a person was to make spinach a regular part of their diet? Would it improve the body's ability to challenge the disease? Would this slow its progress and make a way for the patient to win? The publication **CURRENT MEDICINAL CHEMISTRY** states that the glycolipid in spinach might be a potent anti-tumor compound and may be a healthy food substance with anti-tumor activity.

There are a few cautions to regularly consuming large amounts of spinach. It contains a substantial amount of vitamin K, which is important for blood clotting. If you are on blood thinners, talk with your doctor. Spinach may lower blood sugar levels, so it is necessary to monitor blood sugar levels if you are taking diabetes medications. As a good source of calcium, it may cause hard crystals to form in the kidneys, worsening kidney disease. For some, they may have an allergy to it or some of the environmental companions that accompany them, like certain molds.

Another super green food offering many flavonoids in its leafy greens is kale. For some people, it may be more demanding on the digestive system. Yet, it contains an array of potent flavonoids and carotenoids, including approximately 23 milligrams of quercetin per about 1.5 cup serving of chopped raw kale. Reliable studies show a link between quercetin and its influence on the body's ability to counter cancer cell growth actively.

During the digestion process, isothiocyanates compounds found in these veggies are released into the body, where they can work to fight tumor growth and block its spread. Research has found a relationship between the carotenoids in dark green leafy vegetables, acting to oppose free radicals, preventing them from damaging and combat carcinogenic activity.

Popular in salads is arugula. Its lighter flavor can combine with kale to offset the bitter taste associate with kale. Add some spinach, other veggies, and you have a cancer fighting formula. Arugula is well known in the wholistic health field for its anti-cancer benefits. It is recognized as being amongst the highest of the brassicas veggies for its cancer fighting potential. Researchers contribute arugula's capability to battle mutant cells to a high concentration of glucosinolates, reported to stimulate self-destruction of malignant cells, as well as act as an effective cellular detoxifier to protect cells from damage that may lead to various cancers.

There are several human studies linking the reduction of a number of possible cancers, like prostate, colon, breast, lung, and others, to a high intake of leafy greens. They contain a variety of antioxidants, including kaempferol and quercetin, which have polyphenol anti-oxidants, and are associated with anti-inflammatory properties. Epidemiological studies indicate a relationship between a reduction in cancer and the intake of kaempferol. It appears kaempferol inhibits the ability of cancer cells to duplicate and signal cancer cells to induce apoptosis.

Though some of these studies single out specific compounds as being very effective, the greatest results come as a synergistic effect because of the consumption of the vegetable(s) itself. More data is necessary in humans to further understand how and what compounds have the most benefits. However, sufficient evidence exists to acknowledge the value of leafy greens like spinach, kale, arugula, and others into your regular diet. It just takes a couple of handfuls a day as a part of your regular meals, as a positive step in an integrative approach to cancer care.

You may ask, "What if I don't want to eat salad all the time."

Healthy homemade juices are not difficult to make and enable you to consume more nourishing foods. All you need is a blender. Start with your chosen greens, other vegetables and/or fruit, and maybe some plain yogurt, if you desire a creamy drink, and add liquid. I use green tea for an extra punch of phytonutrients. Blend and drink. Drinking it with all the pulp from the ingredients, you gain the benefit of all the fiber along with the nutrients. But if you find it hard to swallow, then run it through a strainer and it will be more like the consistency of juice.

Bon appétit.

Veggies of the Cross

Regarding nutrient-dense foods, cruciferous vegetables are one of the most valuable. This family of plants essentially encompasses the cabbage family of vegetables. Brussels sprouts, cauliflower, and broccoli are a few better-known members of this family. Rich in many polyphenols, vitamins, and compounds, these veggies provide the body with powerful tools to defend against cancer.

If you are like me, you may be wondering why they are called cruciferous. It comes from our friends, the botanists, who group these plants within the family Criciferae, meaning cross. Within their leaves is the appearance of a cross. For the curious mind who needs to know, there it is.

Broccoli, Brussels sprouts, and other cruciferous vegetables are high in glucaric acids. These compounds are found in many fruits and vegetables and promote normal cellular function. An article in **Cancer Therapies** conveys that preliminary testing indicates that eating foods high in glucaric acid may assist in preventing some forms of cancer, such as prostate and breast cancer.

Cruciferous vegetables may also be called Brassica, including cauliflower, kale, collard greens, arugula, cabbage, and others. These are rich in the nutrients of carotenoids, vitamins C, K, and B vitamin folate, along with minerals, while being a good source of fiber. The cancer-fighting abilities of these vegetables are well documented. Their cancer-combating properties come from glucosinolates, which, during digestion, release isothiocyanates and indoles, phytochemicals linked to lower risk of cancer by reducing inflammation.

Glucosinolates may also trigger the production of enzymes within the body, associated with the deactivation of carcinogens and decreasing metastasis. It is worth noting that it seems to alert genes that stimulate the self-destruction of cancer cells and suppress tumor growth. The **National Cancer Institute** has found that glucosinolates' bioactive compounds are particularly effective against colon, stomach, prostate, breast, bladder, liver, and lung cancers.

Laboratory testing identified these phytochemicals as having chemo preventative effects while protecting against DNA damage to cells, helping the deactivation of carcinogens and inducing apoptosis and anti-inflammatory properties. Along with these activities is the capacity to influence angiogenesis by reducing blood vessel development that feeds a colony of malignant cells, inhibiting the spread and growth of cancer cells.

Several case studies identified a specific gene that encodes glutathione, known as the body's "master detoxifier," to be influenced by the consumption of this family of vegetables. Glutathione (GST) is a complex family of enzymes that play a crucial role in detoxifying the body. They are naturally occurring in this nutrient-dense family of vegetables. GST breaks down for elimination through urination, which influences and removes environmental carcinogens like pollutants and pesticides from the individual. In addition, it acts as antioxidants and anti-inflammatories—all help control or weed out cancer cells.

These glucosinolates appear in relatively high concentrations in all cruciferous vegetables, along with other valuable cancer-fighting nutrients. I include as many of these foods in my weekly diet to gain any advantage possible. Nurturing the microbiome with a powerhouse of phytocompounds can help protect and assist the immune system in combating all diseases.

Beets Me

We often hear about beet juice and beet powder and their ability to boost nitric oxide. What is missing is the role beets can play in reducing the spread of cancer in the body. Information indicates the beetroot is effective in controlling growth of cancers in the lungs, breast, pancreas, prostate, stomach, and brain. Attribute this to the high concentration of betalains, a powerful antioxidant. It gets credit for the ability to hinder tumor cell division. **Howard University**, a research university in Washington, DC, established that the forms of betalains in beets, especially betacyanin, slowed the growth of prostate and breast cancer cells.

Betanin, responsible for beets' deep red color, is shown to aid in detoxification, liver functions, and overall cellular operations within the body. It may be an important part of the cytotoxic effect exhibited by the beetroot extract with breast and prostate cancer cell research in lab experiments. The journal of **PHYTOTHERAPY RESEARCH** analyzed the potent antioxidants of Betanin and isobetanin extracts from beets as a part of a treatment regimen. The conclusion was that the combination offered a synergistic relationship that inhibited the spread of cancer cells and reduced their viability.

There is accumulating evidence identifying betanin as an anti-inflammatory. Laboratory research has determined that it activates a protein that may play a role in regulating gene expression of the master regulator of the antioxidant system. It lies dormant in our cells until called into action; it then binds to antioxidant response elements, activating a battery of detoxifying responses to oxidative disruptors caused by inflammation. This activity is critical for cell protection, survivability, and cancer prevention, and to balanced body chemistry.

Beets are high in dietary nitrates. **THE WORLD CANCER RESEARCH FOUNDATION** recognizes nitrate rich foods as having cancer-fighting properties. They appear to be particularly effective against cancers of the stomach, larynx, pharynx, mouth, and esophagus. The **BRITISH JOURNAL of PHARMACOLOGY** also acknowledged that nitrate rich food offers benefits to overcoming cancer. There are stories of the beneficial nature of vegetable juice, including beetroot. I want to emphasize that positive results are best achieved by an integrative approach that encompasses diet, exercise, lifestyle, and oncology care.

Consideration has to be paid to the fact that beetroot is high in sugar and arginine. It is well established that sugar can contribute to the spread or growth of a mass of mutated cells, while arginine stimulates blood vessel formation, which can feed that growth. The question then becomes, should a person with cancer consume beets? That is a valid question and one to be discussed with your integrative medicine practitioner. The short answer may be to avoid them.

Since they contain some health promoting advantages like aiding in detoxification and supporting liver health, both of which are important when you receive chemotherapy, this makes them helpful. Their relevance as an antioxidant and having anti-inflammatory capabilities earns them a part of a purposefully healthy life. Combine those attributes with the research of betanin/isobetanin combination significantly decreasing the spread of cancer cells and their viability, along with evidence that consuming them may reduce certain side effects of chemotherapy, particularly involving doxorubicin/ Adriamycin. One may want to consider supplementing with beetroot fiber/pectin instead of as food.

That's RAD

The isothiocyanates in radishes have demonstrated the ability to purge the body of cancer agents and influence the genetics of mutant cells, leading to cell death in some cancer cell groups. Preventing them from copying themselves, thereby, stopping the development of tumors. **FOOD CHEMISTRY**, a respected peer-reviewed scientific journal, published a study comparing different vegetables and their ability to reduce cancer growth. Researchers found radishes were over 95% effective in stopping the growth of tumors in the stomach and breast. Much of the credit for this powerful root vegetable is the isothiocyanates, plus its ample supply of other phenolic compounds such as catechins, pyrogallol, and vanillic acid.

Chemotherapy uses powerful chemicals, poisons, that kill cells, ideally targeting faster growing ones like cancer, over normal regeneration of healthy cells. It is an effective treatment for many types of cancers, yet it has side effects. Medications are broken down by the liver, so your liver enzymes are regularly tested by a healthcare provider during and after treatment. This is to alert them to abnormalities that may lead to liver damage. Regular detoxification through diet is a good way of helping to remove contaminates from our body that leads to liver damage.

Radishes are good for the digestive system and assist in detoxification, helping the body to cleanse the blood and remove toxins and other waste products. They possess the characteristic ability to assist in the manufacturing of bile by the gall bladder, used for digestion and the elimination of waste products, including dead red blood cells from the body. Lab tests have demonstrated that radishes contain compounds that can aid in defending the liver and gall bladder against environmental pollution, and regular consumption of them can improve liver health. Aside from being excellent detoxifiers, they are also rich in vitamin C, folic acid, potassium, fiber, and a number of antioxidants, and they promote anti-inflammatory effects.

Berry Berry Good

Berry interesting and tasty too. Sorry for being silly. I blame it on the chemo effect. Blueberries, strawberries, raspberries, and many other berries, along with cherries, are among the numerous potent types available. From the immune booster elderberry to the less considered cranberry, each has a reputation for some type of medicinal benefit that dates back thousands of years. It is important to be aware that while many of them contain natural occurring compounds that are useful to us, they may also have native chemicals that can make you sick.

Two health enhancing bioactive compounds, which have already been discussed and are common in a variety of berries identified by the **National Institute of Health,** are flavonoids and anthocyanins. Research has verified these to have anti-inflammatory and antioxidant protection. Recent studies have found these substances to be inhibitors of angiogenesis, to provide cells with protection from DNA damage, and to have the ability to induce apoptosis with mutant cells. This observation was confirmed in laboratory tissue studies and human dietary ones using various berry fruits.

Researchers are analyzing flavonoids extensively for their pharmacological effects. Among the readily recognizable flavonoids are anthocyanins. Anthocyanins are what give fruits their distinct pigment and are very prevalent in strawberries, raspberries, blueberries, cranberries, blackcurrants, and others. There is little known about how more than 500 different types interact with the body. For this reason, much of the focus in laboratory research centers around anthocyanin's synergistic effects with the molecular structures within the body.

One of the most recognized flavonoids is resveratrol. For some people, this is a recognizable phytochemical because it is the most fun to consume. Yep, if you are a wine drinker, you may take comfort in knowing it contains resveratrol, a known cancer fighting compound. Dr. David Sinclair, a professor of genetics at **Harvard Medical School**, mentions this in the school's health letter, commenting on resveratrol as helping improve cancer outcomes in laboratory testing.

Nature's npj Precision Oncology, an international peer review journal, refers to resveratrol as a nutraceutical, bioactive compound that can help maintain good health and prevent illness. The journal describes how there is a wealth of information from experiments in the laboratory and that it could be a promising therapeutic agent. Part of the pharmacological action is that resveratrol demonstrates effectiveness in all three stages of carcinogenesis: initiation, promotion, and progress. Research offers the possibilities of a chemo-preventative along with chemotherapeutic effects on cancers. It displays as a promising anti-cancer agent by targeting multiple regulatory pathways, including the promotion of cancer cell death.

Commercially, resveratrol is hyped as a healthy component of red wine, but it is also found in grapes and grape juice, peanuts, blueberries, cranberries, cocoa, pistachios, and other foods. Including these foods as a part of your diet plan will assist in creating a bio-friendly environment within you. However, the reality is the research performed is more inline with quantities found in supplemental forms. By the recommendation of Dr. Keith Block's staff, I began taking 300 mg of supplemental resveratrol daily, along with eating foods with a higher concentration of it. The average glass of red wine contains approximately 1.9 mg of it. Wow! What a party that would be to try and consume that recommended dosage. Now you understand why a supplemental form is the best source of resveratrol.

Blueberries contain high levels of powerful antioxidants, specifically abundant amounts of the cancer fighting phytochemicals of anthocyanins and resveratrol, each of which has been discussed earlier. Blueberries are sometimes referred to as the "king of antioxidant foods." This label comes from its high concentration of compounds that give protection against unstable molecules that can lead to cells becoming cancerous. Their abilities to reduce oxidative stress may carry over to possible prevention of DNA damage. One hundred people involved in a study were given approximately one liter of blueberry juice to drink every day. After one month, there was a 20 percent reduction in cell DNA damage caused by free radicals.

Additionally, blueberries are also a valuable source of vitamin C and manganese. We are all very familiar with vitamin C, but manganese kind of sounds like a disease. Manganese is a micronutrient, essential for the body to perform many functions. It is also a superoxide dismutase (SOD), an antioxidant enzyme important to the body. It converts the most dangerous free radicals into smaller molecules that do not damage the body.

Along with well known citrus fruits like oranges, strawberries are a worthy source of vitamin C. It is important that we consume plenty of foods providing this essential nutrient because the body is unable to produce it on its own. One cup of strawberries provides 150 percent of the daily requirements of vitamin C. Supporting the body with ample amounts of this vitamin, aids in the rebuilding of damaged tissue and bones that often occurs during cancer treatments. Be sure to talk with your oncologist, since there is the possibility that it may hinder chemotherapy effectiveness.

Pelargonidin, another antioxidant that is prevalent in strawberries and other berries, has been demonstrated in lab experiments to block tumor growth along with promoting good liver health. When used in extract form, it was shown to help kill breast cancer cells. Invitro studies also found it to be anticarcinogenic by its effectiveness at battling free radicals. Strawberries also contain the antioxidants lutein and zeathancins, two beneficial compounds that promote good eye health.

Strawberries and other berries contain an extraordinary number of antioxidants, and one of them is ellagic acid. Ellagic acid, which acts as a defense mechanism, is also found in walnuts and pecans and some mushrooms. An article in the journal **Cancer Biology and Medicine**, discusses ellagic acid as exhibiting anticarcinogenic effects by diminishing tumor growth, inducing cancer cell death, blocking inflammation, and other cancer resisting characteristics. Treatments with ellagic acid have been noted as being highly effective in reducing carcinogenesis. This is true even in small doses as you would find in foods like strawberries' ability to reduce inflammation.

Blackberry fruit contains an array of potent phytonutrients as well. These nutrient valuable fruits contribute a plentiful portion of vitamin C. One cup of these wholesome berries has more than 70 percent of the suggested daily requirements of vitamin C. This vitamin plays a significant role in supporting the development of collagen, the major building blocks needed to repair tissue and bones. Blackberries carry the antioxidant anthocyanin, also found in berries such as raspberries, pomegranates, and plums.

Each of the berry fruits pack an ample supply of fiber important to the digestive balance, a major part of the body's immune system. Many of the edible berries have exhibited a chemo preventive response to cancer, predominantly of the intestinal tract, prostate, lung, liver, pancreas, and breast. A variety of these tasty morsels in your diet can compliment conventional cancer treatments and offer potential help to patients with an improved prognosis.

Be fairly warned that berries may carry on them, from the fields, a high concentration of pesticides. The USDA, the governing body for protecting our produce, assures that they are of safe levels. What if you enjoy a lot of them? The body is not designed to filter out these chemicals. If small amounts kill field creatures, might there be a cumulative effect on our bodies? I prefer to consume as little of any chemical that is designed to kill a pesky rascal.

Either way, according to much of the research I've read, making berries a part of your regular diet, regardless of whether they are organic or not, is a valuable asset in your battle with cancer. The natural occurring protective chemicals mentioned, along with many others, contained in berries, make them potent defenders of health and outweighs the possible chemicals that can come with plants sprayed with insecticides or herbicides.

An Apple a Day, or More ...

An increasing number of studies on the common apple promote the eating of apples with a reduced risk of cancer. Pectin, a major dietary fiber in apples, supports the development of gut flora, which is important for protecting colon cells. Also, there is a growing amount of documentation discussing the importance of a healthy gut biome to overall well-being.

Apples contain high concentrations of plant compounds such as antioxidants and triterpenoids, which are in the skin of apples. Triterpenoids exhibit potential chemoprevention and therapeutic effects. Studies conducted at **Cornell University** accredit triterpenoids in apple peels with the anticancer characteristics of lower inflammation, promoting apoptosis, and decreasing the spread of malignant cells. In experiments with laboratory rats being fed a known mammary carcinogenic agent, the group given the human equivalent of one apple a day recorded a 25 percent reduction in tumor occurrence. When supplied with what was equal to three apples a day, there was a 61 percent decrease in the incidence of tumors.

Multiple studies provide an argument for the positive effects of the consumption of apples with their peel. Doctor Michael Greger presents the evidence that the phytonutrients contained in the peel of an apple appear to possess the ability to reignite a cancer-suppressing protein called maspin. The basis for his comments is a report in the **Journal of Nutrition and Cancer.**

The researchers bought apples from a nationally recognized food store, ground them, peel included, into a liquid. They then dripped the juice into Petri dishes containing cancer cultures of two types of breast cancer cells, and two separate ones with different malignant prostate cells. During the weeks that the study took place, in each of the four dishes, the cancerous cells died down to a minimal number. There appears to be a positive correlation between consuming apples with the peel and the reduction of tumor size and metastasis.

This is a good time to again bring awareness to eating organic. Apples are one of the highly exposed fruits to toxic chemicals. Avoiding any carcinogens is obviously advantageous to our well-being. If you are unable to go organic, eating large amounts of fruits and vegetables is better than not consuming them. An additional option is to blend organic apple peel powder with other fruits or vegetables, for flavorful smoothies.

Another one of the hidden gems contained in an apple is glucaric acid. This chemical compound is naturally occurring in the body and is found in apples, citrus fruits, and a number of cruciferous vegetables. Foods high in glucaric acid may help reduce cancer risks as it is an integral part of cleansing the body of contaminates.

The liver is your body's detoxifying organ, and it is there that it attaches toxins to glucuronic acid. From the liver, these toxins go to the small intestines to be excreted from the body as a part of a protective process. Natural occurring bacteria in the digestive tract produce an enzyme called beta-glucuronidase and appears to be more prevalent when there is an absence of higher amounts of fiber. If there is a high level of this enzyme present in the gut, it can break the bond between glucuronic acid and the toxins sent by the liver to be removed from the body. When this happens, the contaminant can be reabsorbed into the body. This is not good.

Appearing in **Alternative Medicine Review**, glucaric acid's ability to inhibit the enzyme beta-glucuronidase, could be constructive in reducing hormone dependent cancers of the prostate, breast, and colon. Hormones that have reached the end of their useful life or exist in overabundance are attached to glucaric acid, like toxins, to be excreted from the body. To help maintain an appropriate balance of valuable microbes in the digestive tract, it is crucial to eat high fiber foods like apples.

It appears that the old adage, "An apple a day helps keep the doctor away," is not without a solid foundation. A note: Glucaric acid is available as a supplement, but check with your doctor, because it can possibly enhance or decrease some drugs' effectiveness.

Fungus Among Us

One food group I think is often overlooked is fungi. Now doesn't that sound appetizing? If you travel outside the United States, that is what you will find on the menu, while here in the U.S., we try to make it more appetizing, so we call them mushrooms, Possibly the most overlooked of the super foods. They may be the largest organism on the earth because of their mycelium living beneath the surface. Within this group are numerous types of edible ones, offering tremendous potential for what ails us.

Historically, in eastern medicine, mushrooms have been acknowledged for their healing and immunostimulant properties for thousands of years. Science has established that their functional benefits may stem from the fact that we share roughly between 50 and 85 percent, depending on the mushroom, of our genetic makeup with these fungi. It is not exactly pleasant to imagine ourselves as having aspects in common with a thing that grows in poop, yet that is what makes their nutrients so bioavailable. Not the poop but the common genetics.

Bioavailability is just a scientific way of saying that the beneficial compounds in mushrooms are efficiently absorbed and stand a better chance of being effective in the human body. The defense mechanism these fungi use to protect and flourish in their environment may also aid us. Is it a wonder that as much as 40 percent of pharmaceuticals currently on the market contain some type of mushroom extract?

Some mushrooms that carry the medicinal label for improved health are shiitake, maitake, cordyceps, lion's mane, and oyster mushrooms. These fungi contain polysaccharides, important to cellular communications, that stimulate the immune system. They do this by providing us with vital nutrients like B vitamins, selenium, copper, glutathione, fiber, and amino acids, which are some of their valuable contributions to a healthy body. In studies involving the testing of mushrooms and individuals, an increase in the number of immune cells was noted, along with multiplying the activity of such cells in patients given mushroom extract.

Both phytochemicals and antioxidants exist in abundance in mushrooms. Even the common button mushroom tops the antioxidant levels found in well known fruits and vegetables such as tomatoes and green peppers. This intense concentration of health promoting compounds may play a role in improving immune function and even "suppressing the growth and reproduction of certain cancer cells," says Harry Marsales, a researcher at the **University at Buffalo's Department of Exercise and Nutrition.**

The application of phytochemicals derived from mushrooms has been used to prevent the recurrence of some cancers in Japan for generations. In one case, patients who underwent radiation therapy for endometrial and cervical cancer were given mushroom extract. Observations exhibit that there were three times fewer cancer cells than those who were not provided with them.

In an examination of 185 patients with advanced stage lung cancer, who received radiation treatments and were given mushroom extract, as compared to those who did not receive it, there was a 400 percent increase in survival rates after five years for those who got the additional supplement. Similar increases in the effectiveness were noticed also with chemotherapy treatment. The understanding is because it arrests the spread of malignancies, while the body's own immune systems fight cancer cells.

One of the more researched compounds in mushrooms is beta-glucans. This potent polysaccharide consists of numerous molecules bonded together and are component parts of bacteria and fungi. They stimulate the immune system by enhancing the function of our natural killer (NK) cells, T-cells, macrophages, and other white blood cells, improving the body's ability to fight disease producing organisms, engulfing microbes, cancer cells, and any other things that do not possess the proper protein profile that makes up a healthy cell.

It is critical to note that not all mushrooms are edible. Some contain compounds that are toxic, causing poisoning, allergic reactions, infections, and, in worst cases, death. Unless you are a highly trained mycologist, a person who studies fungi, the Mushroom Council says to consume only mushrooms purchased through a trusted retail outlet. Poisonous ones may resemble edible mushrooms. A safer and more potent option is to purchase extracts from health food stores and online.

Shiitakes may be the best known of the more exotic mushrooms. In the ancient Orient, they were considered the food of the aristocracy. They boost the immune system by supporting an increase in white blood cell production. Additionally, they possess anti-inflammatory properties and are rich in selenium, which is connected with a lower risk of certain cancers, while also protecting cell DNA and destroying some cancer cells.

Reishi mushrooms have become popular through investigations that identify their effectiveness in strengthening the immune system. A study published in **Food & Function**, a journal linking food chemistry and its relationship to health, chronicled the results of laboratory testing of reishi mushrooms and their relationship to immune function. These fungi exhibit a propensity to alter inflammation pathways and have positive effects on the immune system.

Next is the "king of mushrooms," the maitake. These beneficial morsels are acclaimed by Asian medicine as an adaptogen, or herbal pharmaceutical, that help oppose the impact of stress on the body and mind. They are renowned for their rich beta-glucan content. The journal **Food Chemistry** posts that fractionalized compounds from maitakes, activate cytotoxic lymphocytes like NK-cells and T-cells, known to attack cancer cells.

Considered to be a protector of the liver, an excellent detoxifier when consumed regularly, the turkey tail mushroom also fights inflammation. Their predominant capacity to heighten immune function puts them in the super food category. The polysaccharides found in this mushroom are potent immunosupportive compounds that help stimulate white blood cells to protect the body against various pathogens.

When looking for a food loaded with vitamins, minerals, and antioxidants, chaga mushrooms rank high in that class. These nutrient dense goodies contain the complex B vitamins, vitamin D, and potassium, vital to cell functions; the cell building blocks amino acids, copper and iron, which are important to blood cells; zinc, critical to the body's defenses; selenium, a contributor to the development of glutathione; and magnesium and calcium.

A study cited by registered dietitian Beth Czerwony, RD, of **The Cleveland Clinic**, observed that the continuous intake of an extract from the chaga mushroom promoted the suppression of some cancer types. The mechanism that causes this effect of cancer prevention is not yet understood. While these findings are not conclusive, and further research is needed, incorporating extracts from this tree fungus as a part of a personal routine may be beneficial.

One of the more popular culinary mushrooms for its light taste is the chanterelles. Like the other mushrooms, they pack tremendous nutritional value. Also present in this fungus is the polysaccharide chitin, important for cell development, stimulating the immune system, reducing inflammation and oxidative stress, and lowering the risk of certain cancers.

Chanterelles value in promoting good health is overlooked in contemporary medicine. In traditional healing practices, they were used for the content of phenolic acids, giving the body a more vigorous immune response through the presence of antioxidants and anti-inflammatory properties. Though research is limited, some laboratory studies have shown that an extract from these mushrooms provides protection against DNA damaging substances.

Also, one of the anticancer properties found in chanterelles and other mushrooms is a naturally occurring chemical compound called lentinan. **The Memorial Sloan Kettering Cancer Center** reports this beta-glucan is not a cancer cell killer by itself, but a few human studies demonstrate that it seems to enhance the immune system by intensifying T-helper cell functions and other killer cells of the immune system, possibly slowing the progression of tumors. The increased value of lentinan as a chemotherapeutic is when it is used in combination with ongoing conventional treatments. Several clinical trials indicate an increase in the effectiveness of some chemotherapy treatments.

It is important to remember that it is not a one-time event. Like all of the fares discussed, they must become a steady component in preparing meals. Medicinal value comes from the regular consumption of these relevant bites of goodness. If you are currently striving to win the cancer crusade, then you'll need more concentrated forms of these hidden treasures.

The strategy then turns the focus to using the more potent extracts or tinctures. Retrieving the beneficial properties available in these supporting elixirs is done differently, with each process capturing specific compounds. Extracts are generally considered to possess a greater concentration of the significant compounds helpful in the cancer battle, but not necessarily all the same concentrations. For instance, the distillation for creating an extract pulls more beta-glucans from the mushrooms than the process used for a tincture, which provides a higher concentration of triterpenoids, potential anti-cancer agents against colon cancer.

With the explosion of supplements, finding functional mushroom compounds in a tincture or powder form has become easier. Both forms can be added to drinks, used in meal preparations, or simply taken as a tablet, all of which appear to be effective. Powders and tinctures are the best way to get the optimum medicinal content from these compounds. Yet, it is still advantageous to include whole mushrooms as a regular part of meal planning.

It is important to keep your doctors informed as to all supplemental steps towards promoting thriving health, and this is especially true with mushrooms. So be sure to ask if there is any conflict with any pharmaceuticals. Generally, medicinal mushrooms are safe for most people when recommended dosages are followed, but there may be possible side effects that must be considered.

DO NOT try functional mushrooms if you have a sensitivity or allergy to any mushroom or plants having spores. Everyone's chemistry is unique to themselves. Be observant of changes physically and in mood, both positive or negative, and take appropriate action. If you feel any sort of discomfort or irritation, **STOP**. Having a functional health practitioner who is knowledgeable in medicinal fungi science as a part of your wellness team, can aid in making informed decisions. I am emphasizing, this book is not to be considered expert. It is only a transfer of information from other sources related to the topic of fungi and their possible health benefits.

This is Nuts

Nuts are a valuable group of whole foods to include in your diet to help maintain a healthier lifestyle. That is, of course, unless you have an allergy to these packages of nutrition; then they can be life-threatening. They are a good source of quality protein, vitamins, and minerals.

All nuts are known for having high levels of beneficial fats, and many contain valuable phytonutrients and antioxidants that have been linked to good cardiovascular health, along with an association to diminished possibilities of some cancers. A variety of polyphenols can be found in tree nuts. Among them are anthocyanins and ellagitannins and lignans, linked to lowering the risk of breast cancer, and naphthoquinones. As stated in **BMC**, a journal that publishes peer reviewed reports, "Naphthoquinones ... have garnered much attention in the scientific community due to their pharmacological properties, among them anticancer action and potential therapeutic significance." Then there are stilbenes, which have been accredited with acting as cancer preventatives by their anti-inflammatory, antioxidant, and cell death activation in animal studies.

This groups them in the superfood category, but without the price tag that may accompany other high-level edibles. It doesn't take a lot of them to either. A mere handful a day packs enough nutrients to have a positive affect. As with all food, a variety will give the greatest return on your nutritional investment.

The arrangement of the following doesn't necessarily imply the order of value. They are organized relative to the frequency of their appearance in my search.

First are walnuts. When talking with health and nutrition experts and reading articles on the topic of nuts, walnuts is often on the top of the list. They are a good source of plant-based omega-3 fatty acids. Information on this nutrient appears to be more readily available than any other I've found. The focus on its healthiness will be centered on combating cancer; omega-3 fatty acids are good for coronary health and positive brain function.

Studies have associated the consumption of foods such as walnuts, containing high concentrations of omega-3s, to a lower risk of some cancers, specifically breast, prostate, and colon cancers. Disclosed in the **Journal of Medicinal Food**, an 18-week examination of animals fed a diet high in walnuts determined the ability to slow the growth of prostate cancer. Review of the findings noted the decline in the hormone IGF-1, which has been associated with both prostate and breast cancers.

Colorectal cancer is a fierce disease and may be on the rise. In addition to early screening for the disease, changing diet to include more fiber, found in nuts, can make it one the most preventable ones. A **Harvard Medical School** study determined a 27% reduction in the rate of colorectal tumor growth among mice fed walnuts. Their ability to significantly diminish tumor angiogenesis needed for cancer to grow, is believed to be the contributing mechanism.

Joe Vinson, Ph.D., a researcher at The **University of Scranton in Pennsylvania**, established that walnuts possess a content of antioxidants between 2 and 15 times more powerful than vitamin E itself. Since they are mostly eaten raw, the antioxidants quality and quantity are preserved as compared to roasted ones. All it takes is a handful a day to gain the advantages of this potent healthy snack.

Another nut packing a nutritional shot to body chemistry are hazelnuts. They are commonly used for their sweet flavor in chocolate making, giving me a good excuse to eat more chocolate. These filberts, as they are sometimes referred to, are exceptionally dense in their nutritional profile and possess significant levels of antioxidants, making them amongst the top in oxygen radical absorption capacity (ORAC). Wrapped within these little power houses are flavonoids, a subgroup of polyphenols that provide amongst the highest concentration of any of the tree nuts. These phytonutrients are capable of supplying free radical protection up to 50 times greater than vitamin E and 20 times higher than vitamin C. The high levels of antioxidants in hazelnuts earns them a place in the superfood grouping when it comes to cancer fighting. To get the most concentration of antioxidants, eat hazelnuts with the skins still on.

A one-ounce serving of hazelnuts contains about 86 percent of the daily requirement of manganese, a trace mineral vital to bodily functions and bone formation. Research published in the **Journal of Inorganic Biochemistry** references experiments conducted with manganese at a **University in China,** finding that a complex of manganese is "active against cancer cells."

Also, with a one-ounce serving of hazelnuts, you get 24 percent of the needed copper crucial to the body's regular operations, including the immune system. In scientific experiments, there is evidence of copper oxide playing a role of inhibiting the growth of pancreatic tumor cells by contributing to the apoptosis of cancer stem cells in laboratory cultures. There is also evidence of copper inclusion in cancer therapeutics arresting the proliferation of colon cancer cells. This essential trace mineral is needed to promote healthy cell activities.

Supplementation is not suggested since high levels of it may increase the possibility of some types of cancer.

One of my favorite plant proteins is almonds. Though classified as a tree nut, it is actually the seed of a fruit related to the peach. They are potent in nutrition, antioxidants, vitamins, and minerals, helping protect against the damaging effects of oxidative stress that contribute to inflammation. To get the most benefit from these robust substances that, according to the **Mayo Clinic**, "may play a role in protecting your cells from free radicals," you must eat almonds with the brown skins on, where most of these compounds are found.

The polyphenols in almonds were discovered to be very accessible to the body, making them easily metabolized by enzymes and intestinal flora. A major antioxidant in them is tocopherol, which is found in vitamin E. A one-ounce serving (28.4 grams) provides about 37 percent of the required intake of this protective nutrient. An excerpt from the **New England Journal of Medicine** reported a link between the intake of vitamin E with lower rates of cancer and other chronic conditions like coronary heart disease. This, along with other antioxidants in almonds, can assist in the prevention of cell damage caused by oxidation.

An examination of murine studies published in **Cancer Letters**, found a correlation with the reduction of colon cancer cells and the consumption of almonds. Combined with observational research reported in the **American Society of Clinical Oncology**, of over 800 colorectal patients, established that those who ate almonds along with other tree nuts weekly, "...had a 42 percent lower chance of cancer recurrence and 57 percent lower chance of death than those who did not eat nuts."

Another tree nut containing beneficial cancer fighting nutrients are Brazil nuts. Native to the Amazon rainforest, these nuts are a terrific source for the trace element selenium, a component part of selenoproteins. These proteins are essential to the body, playing an important role in immune response, the process of promoting cell viability, along with other important roles. This mineral is only found in certain foods like eggs, seafood, seeds, and others, with Brazil nuts having one the highest concentrations of it.

Low levels of selenium have been associated with a number of deficiencies, including immune system disfunction, cognitive issues, and fatigue, to name a few. Clinical trials on raised blood levels of selenium have demonstrated an improvement with thyroid problems, which may occur from some cancer therapies, and an increase of the enzyme glutathione peroxidase, whose main role is protecting the body from oxidative stress.

Selenium's effective antioxidant properties, its capacity to influence apoptosis, immune and hormonal systems, and positive impact on DNA repair, provides some clout as a valuable mineral in the prevention of cancer. A review of research that tracks the patterns and effects of disease and the benefits of intermediaries on health care, indicates that people with the highest intake of selenium had a 31 percent lower risk of some cancers, and in men, a decreased prospect of prostate cancer by 22 percent.

Of the most favored nuts, cashews are near the top of the list. These tasty snacks contain an array of valuable nutrients associated with good health. A part of their nourishing composition includes vitamin K, important to blood clotting; an abundance of thiamine, needed for energy; vitamin B6 and zinc for supporting the immune system;

phosphorus for strong bones; and iron for red blood cell development to carry oxygen in the body. They are a good source of healthy fats and protein, as well as providing the minerals of copper, magnesium, and manganese, along with being a fiber rich food.

As with many tree nuts, cashews contain an array of phytochemical compounds associated with anti-inflammatory, free radical fighting antioxidants. Some of these chemical compositions create anti-proliferation effects with tumor cells, chemo preventative agents, along with other possible interventions. One of their honorable attributes is an anti-cancer catechol, a small molecule that has demonstrated an ability to inhibit the growth of lung cancer cells, while not damaging healthy ones.

Raw cashews may contain a poisonous substance called urushiol that may have seeped through from the shell. Separating them from the shell, then roasting, eliminates the urushiol, making them safe to eat. Additionally, some research indicates that roasted cashews appear to promote greater antioxidant activities. Though it is easy to roast them at home, it's easier to choose the roasted ones when shopping. Look for dry roasted, as they are free of less healthy fats.

The delicate and almost sweet taste of pecans makes them a desirable leader in the nut family. Within the nut group, they are also a major contributor of over 19 vitamins and minerals, with significant levels of the antioxidant vitamin E. They contribute considerable amounts of magnesium, calcium, and potassium, all necessary minerals for a well functioning body. Include a handful a day in your diet as a way to boost protein and fiber. Add to it their certification by the American Heart Association as "heart-healthy," and now we're talking superfood.

Pecan's rich magnesium content delivers an anti-inflammatory shot. Small amounts of inflammation are important for the body's natural defenses to repair damaged cells, along with oxidative stress, but too much can lead to cancer. Pecans act as a natural anti-inflammatory; controlling it reduces the possibility of cell mutations caused by this chronic condition, thereby in one way lessening the chance of altered cells becoming cancerous.

They are packets of minerals including copper. An individual's lack of copper may lead to the presence of fewer white blood cells necessary for fighting pathogens that invade the body from injury and the environment. The **Linus Pauling Institute at Oregon State University** reports that copper may manage the formation of chemical compounds from amino acids within the body. These proteins may inhibit or enhance the process by which a strand of DNA may duplicate, helping to reduce contributors of oxidative stress caused by an imbalance between free radicals and antioxidants, that leads to chronic diseases like cancer.

Pecans also contain a number of other agents with possible cancer fighting abilities. Ellagic acid, a naturally occurring tannin compound, is one of those potential agents. Laboratory investigations have studied ellagic acid as an antioxidant and an antimicrobial, and its anti-proliferation properties. Research indicates the possibility it may bind to certain carcinogens that can damage DNA, for removal from the body, thereby acting as a cancer-preventative.

The phytonutrients in nuts and seeds are very bio available to the body, meaning they are easily absorbed. These nutrients have been correlated with interrupting the initiation of, and spread of, numerous pathogenic mechanisms, including those related to cancer.

Observational studies, one appearing in the **British Journal of Cancer**, suggest the possibility of an inverse relationship between tree nut consumption and malignancies, among them pancreatic cancer.

Which if any of the nuts have the greatest return relative to consumption? Dr. Manish Shah, director of **Gastrointestinal Oncology at NY Presbyterian Weil Cornell Medicine Cancer Center**, commented on research on colon cancer and how it is affected by nut consumption. The study appearing in the **Journal of Clinical Oncology** observed the most effective ones were hazelnuts, walnuts, almonds, and pecans.

Like any observational research, it is important to recognize that the data only equates an interrelationship and not necessarily the source of the effect. Many factors can influence the degree to which an action can determine an outcome. A person who eats nuts may also have a tendency to have a healthier lifestyle, eating better quality and nutritious foods.

Epidemiological studies regularly show a strong correlation between a diet rich in fruits and vegetables and a reduced risk of chronic diseases such as cancer. Research indicates that no specific phytonutrient alone can be singled out as optimal. Rather it is synergistic relationship of many fruits and vegetables and their phytonutrients profiles that provide the best offensive to building a healthy body.

Diet is a step towards developing an integrative approach to a balanced, healthy body. To borrow an analogy I once read, imagine a mobile that hangs from the ceiling over a baby's bed, precisely in balance. If one part is pushed or pulled, the whole thing moves.

Gradually, it returns to a state of equilibrium. If a part on one side was removed or was added without consideration of its affect, it throws everything out of balance and the mobile collapses into a state of jumbled material with no balance. That is how the body works.

The gastrointestinal tract plays a key role in the immune system. There is a lot of talk these days about having a healthy gut. That is because the intestinal tract, along with the lymphoid tissue, is responsible for more than 70 percent of our immune functions. Stress from a hectic life, the standard American diet—rich in sugar and saturated fats, while low in fiber—along with high alcohol consumption, gluten, dairy, and select grains, can lead to internal inflammation and damage to the digestive tract.

The intestinal lining covers over 4000 square feet of surface area. A healthy gastrointestinal wall maintains a tight barrier, controlling what it allows into the blood stream while guarding against those things that can harm it. A layer of cells, called the mucosa, lines the interior of the body, protecting it from various pathogens. An unhealthy gut lining may not block toxins, viruses, or bacteria. Allowing them to pass from the digestive tract into the body leads to internal inflammation. This intestinal permeability is sometimes referred to as leaky gut.

Research indicates a leaky gut may trigger internal inflammation and disrupt the balance, possibly leading to problems within the digestive tract and other bodily systems. Studies also indicate that disruptions in gut bacteria and the inflammation from leaky gut may be a player in the development of several common chronic diseases, conceivably autoimmune conditions, and perhaps even mental afflictions.

For decades, holistic, integrative, and functional medicine practitioners have often started balancing the gut microbiota as the initial step to treat chronic conditions. Similarly, ancient medicinal practices and Eastern cultures frequently consider the digestive tract important for healing. Even Western trained doctors commonly change their patients' diets as a step to better health. Having a quality diet and avoiding foods that may be harmful to an individual are two actions a person can take to strengthen the immune system and improve health.

Whether a leaky gut causes the development of other diseases external to the digestive tract, may be controversial among conventionally trained medical personnel. Regardless, much evidence exists to support that eating nutritious food helps suppress inflammation. This can aid in the rebuilding of the mucosal lining and balancing the gut flora. Caution: A side effect of improved dietary practices is more energy, and feeling better physically as well as emotionally.

By the Way ...

The following reviews some foods worthy of inclusion into a cancer-fighting diet while promoting a healthy lifestyle. You have probably heard the term "Eat the rainbow." Brightly colored fruits and vegetables indicate the presence of valuable phytonutrients, vitamins, and minerals. In addition, deep colored fruits and vegetables, like citrus fruits, sweet potatoes, berries, carrots, members of the squash family, and other plant foods, contain the antioxidants carotenoids.

Beta-carotene is one of those carotenoids. It enhances the body's ability to deal with free radicals. Generally overlooked is its ability to improve liver health, function as a detoxifier, and the capacity of it to strengthen the body's immune response and aid in fighting cancers related to the skin, eyes, and some organs. The spectrum of phytonutrients found in many of these incredible edibles also act as antioxidants and protectors of healthy cells.

The **American Institute for Cancer Research** reports that limited laboratory studies found that phytochemicals comparable to those in asparagus can inhibit cancer spread by activating signaling pathways that induce the destruction of abnormal cells. For example, quercetin in asparagus, in companion with its other compounds, influences genes by controlling the expression of those that may enable abnormal cells to develop into cancerous ones, while increasing the expression of cancer-fighting genes. Additionally, the glutathione contained in asparagus may contribute to reducing the spread of cancer cells.

Data involving human testing on the effects of asparagus and cancer risk mostly appears with information by comparing people with a higher dietary vegetable intake, but not singularly by itself. As previously expressed, convincing evidence supports eating higher concentrations of fruits and vegetables contain cancer-fighting phytonutrients like flavonoids, known to act as antioxidants, anti-inflammatories, and enzymes that assist in deactivating carcinogens.

Earlier, there was a discussion about nuts and their benefits. But not to be forgotten are an array of tasty seeds. They have a variety of vital micronutrients, such as calcium, potassium, phosphorus, and magnesium. Seeds worthy of inclusion are chia, hemp, pumpkin, and sunflower, all having favorable fatty acids, which help curtail inflammation, plus they contain a variety of trace minerals. Hemp seeds are a perfect protein because they contain 20 amino acids, including the essential nine that the body cannot produce. Also, they have vital micronutrients like zinc, magnesium, phosphorus, and others. The common sunflower seed possesses the all-important antioxidants valuable to keeping free radicals in check, thus reducing cancer risk. In addition, numerous nourishing trace elements, including copper and selenium, are within those crunchy morsels, along with vitamins E and folate, protein, fiber, and unsaturated fats.

Chemical reactions are continuously taking place in the body, which enables it to perform regular activities to sustain life. These chain reactions require a stimulant called enzymes. Some of these enzymes necessary for the many biochemical responses within the body are proteins. Digestion, muscle movement, levels of energy, and bodily functions rely on these enzymes.

Nuts and seeds are rich in protein, provided allergies are not an issue. In addition, several greens pack many grams of protein in each cup, like green peas, spinach, artichokes, avocados, asparagus, Brussels sprouts, mushrooms, kale, edamame, tofu, legumes, and many others.

The final food I will cover is onions. If an apple a day keeps the doctor away, an onion a day (along with its relative garlic) may keep everyone away. Therefore, you won't catch any illness from them. Thanks for putting up with my silliness. Here are why onions are valuable as an ingredient in cooking many dishes. Beneficial disease-fighting chemicals are present in a variety of onions. Recall the deep color of other fruits and vegetables, representing more or higher concentrations of these valued natural compounds; this pertains to onions also.

Onions are packed with nutrients, including vitamins C and B6, manganese, chromium, and folate, and contain small amounts of other vitamins and minerals, along with a high concentration of sulfur compounds that act as anti-inflammatories and have antimicrobial properties, thereby aiding in boosting the immune system.

They are a good source of quercetin, discussed earlier, known as an antioxidant powerhouse and recognized as reducing inflammation in the body, making onions valuable in lowering the risk of inflammatory diseases like arthritis. In addition, laboratory testing has demonstrated the ability to protect cells against damage that may lead to cancer.

Anthocyanins are responsible for the deep red color of some onions. You may remember this flavonoid is valued as an anti-inflammatory, protects against oxidative stress, and supports healthy DNA to prevent tumor development. In laboratory studies, anthocyanins helped protect against the spread of some cancers while promoting physical health and mental well-being. It is found in various foods such as dark chocolate, red wine, berries, tea, plums, and pomegranate.

The **Journal of Nutrition** reports that the allium family of vegetables, such as onions, contains various bioactive compounds or phytochemicals that can influence bodily functions and inhibit cancer development in some organs. One specific area is the colon. As published in the **Asian-Pacific Journal of Clinical Oncology**, senior author Doctor Zuni Li states, "It is worth noting that in our research, there seems to be a trend: the greater the amount of allium vegetables, the better the protection."

Many foods benefit a healthy lifestyle, and some are best to avoid. A description of the ones to refrain from is primarily in the chapter on the Standard American Diet or SAD. Keep in mind, our bodies evolved to take advantage of food close to its native form. However, some of the manufactured "franken-foods" may not resemble their original form, may lack nutrition, may cause digestive problems, and are difficult for the body to metabolize. Though convenient, recent research indicates that highly processed foods, including refined sugar and oils, grains, packaged meals, and such, may contribute to various physical and mental challenges. In addition, their artificial and manufactured contents are increasingly considered disruptive to the body's microbiome and may contribute to maladies like food allergies.

Eating more organics, avoiding as many processed foods as possible, consuming a variety of natural foods, and focusing on fruits, vegetables, and organic whole grains are positive steps to balancing the digestive environment. As discussed earlier, the gut is the most significant part of the immune system, and it needs to be healthy to fight off illness and prevent other afflictions. To keep it in good condition and strong, eating whole foods while avoiding others is essential to promoting good health. Become a label reader and look at the ingredients, bypassing things like artificial sweeteners, high fructose corn syrup, trans-fats, and those packaged foods where you can't pronounce what's in it. Be wary of fat-free labels; many add extra sugars or chemical additives for the flavor lost from having no fat.

Nutrients, a peer reviewed academic journal, reports a diet rich in plant-based foods consistently links to lower cancer risk. Many researchers contribute this, at least in part, to the phytochemicals found in vegetables, fruits, and other plant foods rich in these protective polyphenols.

By now, you get it. But if you didn't, here is the "Cliff Notes" version. Though there is no single food that would prevent cancer, adopting a diet rich in natural food, and high in fiber, vitamins, and minerals, provides the greatest benefits in preventing some types of cancer by as much as 70 percent. Examination of research supports the concept that a quality diet made up of mostly vegetables and fruits is important for treating, dealing with, and recovering from cancer. A patient's quality of life can be enhanced with healthy plant focused fare, accompanied by good protein sources. I believe it is worth adopting new dining habits to provide yourself with the most significant opportunity of winning.

It's the Little Things

Something extra to do that may increase the effectiveness of your treatments and an anti-cancer diet, is to be sure that you are drinking as pure water as possible. Fortunately, in the Western part of the world, most of the water we drink is free of illness-causing microorganisms like bacteria, and meets federally mandated guidelines that balance the risk between protection from waterborne disease and the consumption of sanitizing chemicals. Most municipal water systems use chlorine as the primary bacteria-controlling agent.

The risk of developing cancer from drinking tap water has never established chlorine as the culprit. There are many investigations into water contamination and cancer-causing agents in the water supply, and there is limited evidence pointing exclusively at chlorine. Most of the studies between water quality and cancer are concentrated in specific geographical areas, looking at the percentage of deaths of people who had cancer in a population. The investigations offered limited support to the hypothesis established in laboratory testing and standards of water disinfectants in municipal water supplies and incidence of various cancers other than those of the colon. However, epidemiological studies, those looking at a population, indicate that the implications of cancer are unconnected to water chlorination and are more likely related to lifestyle issues like smoking or other environmental exposures.

As mentioned, consuming chlorinated water may increase the susceptibility to colon cancer, understandable since the purpose of treating water with it is to kill pathogens like bacteria. I could not find any considerable research on the effects of consuming chlorinated water on gut microbiology. But a study on the consumption of water disinfected by chloramine, a less aggressive alternative to chlorine, disrupted the immune system of laboratory animals. Your digestive system, significant to healthy immune function, needs the proper balance of beneficial bacteria to work properly. Chlorine is indiscriminate. It kills all types of bacteria.

Other agents in drinking water that remain after the purification process, range from industrial farming residual runoffs of fertilizers and pesticides, lead, mercury, pharmaceuticals, and an array of other chemicals, all of which are detrimental to health. Reports as recent as 2020 state that carcinogenic chemicals, ranging from radioactive agents to a family of over 9000 compounds called per-and polyfluoroalky substances (PFAS), including those featured in the movie *Dark Waters*, are in many municipal water supplies.

A growing body of evidence has raised concerns about the potential adverse health effects of PFAS exposure. They are sometimes referred to as "forever chemicals" because they can build up in the body and stay for a long time. Some research suggests a link between high concentrations of PFAS in the body and various cancers, adverse effects on the immune system, liver damage, thyroid disease, obesity, reduced fertility, hormone suppression, delayed mental development in children, and other negative health issues. The U.S. government is beginning to study PFAS and their removal from our water supply, but this may take decades to implement an effective solution.

Well water is often used as the standard of "clean and unaffected by environmental contaminants" when considering the quality of water supplies. However, recently measured groundwater is of concern for the presence of pesticides, industrial solvents, and other synthetic chemicals established as carcinogenic in laboratory studies. Testing reveals that the depth of the aquifer matters. Shallow wells are more susceptible to industrial and rural runoff. Wells 100 feet or deeper appear to have the lowest content of these pollutants. However, they may have a higher content of radium, a radioactive chemical element. So, have your well evaluated for the presence of contaminants and radium.

An alternative is bottled water. As it pertains to chemicals present in the water, plastic bottles may be worse than tap water. Plastic has various chemicals that leach into the water contained within the bottle. The most common is BPA or bisphenol A, which the FDA has banned in baby bottles. Testing of BPA and BPS, a manufacturing substitution for BPA (sneaky rascals), at the **University of Texas Medical Branch at Galveston**, established that concentration levels of less than one part per trillion of these chemicals could obstruct the orderly operation of cell activity. These chemicals can disrupt genetic messaging in cells, proper hormone regulation in our body, and cause congenital disabilities and possibly cancer. One of the ways that can induce the seepage of these compounds from a plastic bottle into its contents is heat. For example, leaving one in a hot car for an undetermined period may release chemicals into the liquid. Another is reheating food in the microwave in plastic food storage containers. It is noticeable as pot marks appear around the container after heating, from the release of chemicals into the contents. If bottled water is your choice, glass is the safest, best option, though more expensive.

What about fluorinated water? Is adding fluoride to municipal supplies an advantage to dental and other health issues? It is a controversial subject. It has raised moments of spirited discussion with a dental professional in my family. Proponents refer to research supporting the reduction of cavities in communities introducing it in the processing water for consumption. However, I have yet to find data on the percentage of cavities in communities without fluoridation, for comparison. This information would be valuable as dental hygiene has uniformly improved across the United States in recent decades.

What is fluoride? Any compound that contains fluorine in its makeup is called fluoride. In a highly concentrated gaseous elemental form, it is dangerous and toxic. **De Gruyter**, a publisher of academic papers, wrote an online article recommending extreme caution in its use. Nevertheless, it's common in industrial applications, and variants are a part of the manufacturing of low-friction plastics in some non-stick cookware, to which a few are now banned.

Calcium fluoride is natural in the environment and, in small amounts, beneficial to people, while sodium fluoride is in dental hygiene products. Neither is what municipalities typically add to their drinking water. According to the **American Water Works Association Standards Committee**, approximately 90 percent of the fluoride used in fluoridation is hexafluorosilicic acid. This manufactured compound is a by-product of the production of phosphate fertilizers. The European Union has banned it as a biocidal or life-destroying substance because of the lack of information that it is safe for human consumption and the environment.

Increasingly, research indicates the potential to cause long-lasting negative effects to a number of bodily functions. The magazine of Harvard's **T.H. CHAN SCHOOL OF PUBLIC HEALTH** reported, "Perhaps most worrisome is preliminary research in laboratory animals, suggesting that high levels of fluoride may be toxic to brain and nerve cells. And human epidemiological studies have identified possible links to learning, memory, and cognition deficits, though most of these studies have focused on populations with fluoride exposures higher than those typically provided by U.S. water supplies." A **U.S. EPA** document has stated, "Concentrations of hexafluorosilicic acid may be present in the gastrointestinal tract after consumption of fluoridated drinking water."

In 2013, a former EPA scientist, J. William Hirzy, Ph.D., and colleagues, petitioned the EPA to discontinue adding hydrofluosilicic acid (HFS or FSA). Their conclusion is derived from studies showing the possible adverse effects on human health. The data suggest that like most chemicals, natural or manufactured, there are limits to their usefulness; in some instances, absolute avoidance is essential. What is needed is a scientific evaluation and epidemiological studies of fluoride, challenging and comparing the human health cost to benefits of it in our water supply.

What is a person to do? Various home filtration options are available. With all the options available, it can be challenging to determine which water filtration system is desirable for you. To help make that choice, the **Environmental Working Group (ewg.org)**, a research and advocacy group working to improve environmental concerns like clean water, offers a water filtering buying guide that you can view online.

We are very fortunate in the Western world to have water free of dangerous pathogens, which is vital to good health. Yet the unknown forms of manufactured waste are scary and require increased demand on the body to rid itself of contaminants. It is crucial to support it with the best possible means of working for you during your fight to win, and not having other impurities to deal with may be an added advantage. The evidence, I believe, justifies a further means of removing undesirable pollutants. Wherever you source your supply, be it unfiltered community, bottled, a well, or a home filtration unit, drinking plenty of water is good for cleansing the body, along with helping increase energy.

A subject of more recent interest in promoting good health is fasting. One thing it does is assist in supporting detoxification. Even when you eat healthy, organic foods, there is still the regular bombardment by external pollutants. When you fast, it can kick in other organs—the skin, respiratory system, digestive tract, kidneys—all a part of detoxifying and eliminating poisons from the body. When the body's purging process becomes overburdened, unwanted contaminants circulate through the bloodstream and are possibly reabsorbed into the tissues, where they may cause health issues. Allowing the body an opportunity to recover by intermittent fasting, maybe a longer one every three months, can encourage better health by cleansing cells and tissues of these toxins. During cancer treatments and recovery, regular fibrous foods, leafy greens, juicing of fresh fruit and vegetables, fasting, and some herbs promote the body's natural detoxifying and elimination process while enabling the body to regenerate.

Though minor in action, each step assists the body with an improved internal environment to battle cancer and aid treatment recovery. Healthy little extras may boost the effectiveness of an anti-cancer diet. As with all the things discussed, the objective is to provide the body's microbiome with the best opportunity to operate more effectively. Whether it be meaningful choices like eliminating particular foods or avoiding exposure to environmental pollutants, each enables nature to be part of the solution, to not fall victim to ill health.

Science is constantly finding new compounds, micronutrients, and phytochemicals across the plant kingdom that are valuable to staying healthy. Therefore, it is insightful to eat a diversified diet of fruits, vegetables, and other plants as a foundation of a healthy lifestyle. In addition, many of these nutrients can work together to help advance an active response to environmental threats and invaders. At the same time, it is creating a balanced biome within us.

Chapter 8

A Spicy Life

"Remember: Life is short.
Break the rules."
– James Dean

Modern science is discovering what was known by ancient medical practitioners for years: Some spices and herbs offer practical benefits. When we think of them, it's usually flavor enhancers, yet they also contain potent polyphenol compounds. As a reminder, polyphenols are naturally occurring chemicals widely found in plants that they use as defenses against disease. The **National Institute of Health** recognizes many spices and herbs as having high levels of phenolics and that they have demonstrated high antioxidant capacity, as well as anti-inflammatory, antimicrobial, and even anti-cancer properties. With these possibilities, spices deserve to be considered part of a healthy integrative approach to cancer therapy.

Studies have shown that some spices and herbal supplements are safe and effective. However, there are those with big claims attached to them, and their effectiveness has yet to be tested or shown to be possibly harmful or toxic to you.

This material is educational in purpose about some common spices and herbs. It is essential to keep your caregiver informed and validate whenever you include these spices and herbs in your daily practices. The intention of this information is integrative in purpose and to be included with conventional therapies, not as a substitute for them.

Allspice

For instance, a study from the **University of Miami** found that ericifolin, a compound derived from allspice, slowed the growth of prostate cancer cells in mice. The dosage used on the mice was equal to about one teaspoon of allspice powder. Considering that cancer of the prostate is the most common cancer for men, other than those of the skin, this may be a valuable spice to work into your diet.

It is summarized to happen by interfering with the androgen receptors. Androgens are a group of hormones, predominantly testosterone, that primarily influence the male reproductive organs. Receptors are the mechanisms by which the body responds appropriately to these androgens, making them essential to genetic expression. Information about a gene is communicated to the correct cells at the appropriate time, in the right quantities, throughout the cells' lives. Scientists are investigating allspice as an interrupter to the unwanted DNA expression and growth of prostate cancer cells by interfering with androgen receptors.

Of course, this examination is in the lab, and more investigation into its possible validity as an effective tool in the fight against cancer is needed. But ericifolin, the compound found in allspice, may be a helpful preventative step and something to include in your diet as a follow-up to treatments for prostate cancer. The **National Institute of Health** considers that if introduced early after treatments, it may not eliminate the reoccurrence but possibly control it to the extent that it poses little threat to life.

Turmeric

If you haven't heard about the excitement surrounding turmeric, it possibly is because you are a newbie to the world of nutrition and the value of using plant-based foods to prevent chronic disease. Health coach and author of the book**,** *The Superfood Alchemy Cookbook*, Jennifer Iserloh says, "There are over 700 medical studies on turmeric," possibly making it the most researched spice out there for medical use.

In India, where it has been used for centuries in cooking, compared to the United States, most cancer rates are much lower**. Saraswati, Ph.D.**, the co-director of **Breast Cancer Programs at John Hopkins**, believes this to be a factor. In research performed there with rats, breast cancer rates were cut in half after introducing turmeric as a part of the equation.

Curcumin, the active compound in turmeric, has inflammation-fighting properties. Researchers are finding that, in some cases, curcumin promotes changes on the molecular level, which may prevent or even treat cancer. At **John Hopkins**, findings are that it helps clear carcinogens before DNA damage occurs, and possibly repairs some damage that has already happened. In addition, lab tests have demonstrated that it can reduce and stop the spread of cancer cells.

Studies at **Rutgers University** have shown that when combined with the compound phenethyl isothiocyanate, which is in foods like broccoli, cauliflower, and other cruciferous vegetables, curcumin may be valuable in treating prostate cancer, along with being helpful to patients of bone, breast, colon, liver, and other types of malignancies. Another investigation said it had "great potential in the prevention of cancer," because curcumin can obstruct cancer cell development in several ways. In addition, some data indicates a boost to the immune system and energy, possibly from lowering bone marrow suppression related to chemotherapy.

The National Institute of Health says there is evidence that curcumin promotes valuable activity against the spread or growth of melanoma, ovarian cancer, lymphoma, and others, including one important to me, leukemia.

Turmeric's curcumin compound packs a powerful punch as if it is too good to be true. There is a lot of hype surrounding it, yet there is supporting evidence from reputable research labs, including **UCLA**, which stated it was an "anti-cancer" agent. Therefore, it is worth including it in cooking and as a supplement. Regardless of how you add it to your daily routine, be sure to include pepper and some fat when cooking with it to increase absorption by the body.

Garlic

Though I've listed garlic as a spice, it is a vegetable and belongs to the allium class of bulb-shaped plants, including onions, chives, leeks, and scallions. In addition to sulfur, garlic contains flavonoids and selenium, which may benefit health. Furthermore, additional valuable compounds, like oligosaccharides, are known to strengthen the immune system and contribute to improved gut microbiome.

When speaking of garlic, many of us relate the aromatic herb to the delicious Italian dishes and flavorful bread that often accompanies it, as well as the smells of Asian cooking or memories of favorite family recipes that contain it as an ingredient. For some, it's the fragrant odor that may follow, coming from those who have consumed it, which is what possibly keeps the vampires away. Garlic is perhaps one of the best-known taste enhancers in cooking across many cultures. You may not know that some traditional societies realize it as a valuable medicinal herb.

Its folklore as a booster of health and complex phytochemistry has made it one of the more looked-at herbs for strengthening the immune system. More than 2000 research papers have focused on garlic and its effective anti-cancer agents. The active compound in garlic that gives us a lovely scent after its consumption has been the most studied and, discovered to have the greatest benefit, is a sulfur compound called allicin.

As reported in the **European Journal of Pharmacology**, allicin can inhibit the increase of cancer cells of human origin as examined in laboratory murine animals. While helping to control the growth of mutated cells, observation also shows it affects the destruction of the nucleus of such cells, thereby disrupting their DNA-building structure, leading to the death of cancerous cells. Research recognizes allicin as a mechanism for the basis of this anti-proliferation effect.

Organosulfur, derived from allicin, helps to reduce the expression and activation of multiple stimulatory proteins needed for cancer cell development, as reported in the **British Journal of Urology International**, a peer-reviewed medical journal; at the same time, targeting many of the hallmarks of cancer growth, proliferation, and metastasis, generational cell response from environmental stressors, to name a few. **The National Institute of Health** reported that garlic-derived compounds reduce the development of cancer cells by mobilizing enzymes that detoxify carcinogens, demonstrate the ability to suppress the growth of cancer cells, and promote the death of various other types of malignancies.

Garlic's complex phytochemical makeup includes multiple vitamins and minerals. These range from significant percentages of thiamine, vitamin B6, and vitamin C, including a good source of calcium, phosphorus, manganese, and selenium minerals. Each of these contributes to a healthy body and plays a role in your striving to create a more effective immune system. It may be one of the most valuable spices and is readily available to use as a part of an integrative dietary approach to standing up to cancer.

Population studies show a strong association between high consumption of allium-related foods and lower risk of colon, stomach, esophagus, and pancreas cancers. Specifically, the **European Prospective Investigation into Cancer and Nutrition (EPIC)** has an active study into how diet affects cancer, indicating that an increased intake of these vegetables has a connection to a lower risk of digestive-related cancers. Why might these ingredients lower cancer risks? Though the studies are observational, with no definitive explanation of the anti-cancer mechanism, researchers believe the answer lies in the flavonoids and organosulfur compounds formed by allicin.

According to Dr. Lina Mu, an associate professor of epidemiology and environmental health at the **University of Buffalo**, the various sulfur compounds in onions and garlic have anti-carcinogenic effects in animal and human studies. Adding to it, as cited in the **Asia-Pacific Journal of Clinical Oncology**, Dr. Zhi Li says, "It is worth noting that in our research, there seems to be a trend: The greater the number of allium vegetables, the better the protection."

Capsaicin

If you like hot flavorful food, you're probably familiar with this spicy addition to cooking. Capsaicin gives cayenne pepper its zing or kick, enjoyed by some in chili and contained in hot peppers. These contain the highest capsaicin content of approximately 198,000 parts per million. Though found in sweet or bell peppers, the composition is much lower at 4000 parts per million.

The National Institute of Health has published information on the inhibitory potential of capsaicin in tumor development, describing it as possessing anti-mutagenic and anti-carcinogenic properties or the ability to prevent the growth of cancer cells. Many lab models report evidence of preventative as well as therapeutic benefit of capsaicin, by inducing the death of mutated cells. Apoptosis was generated and observed during testing on malignant cells in the linings of organs, breast, and prostate, influencing the viability of these cancer stem cells and others while enhancing the effect of therapeutic agents in some cancer treatments.

As published in the **International Journal of Cancer Research and Treatment**, capsaicin altered the expression of several genes involved in cancer cell survival. It is considered effective in arresting the growth of malignant cells, angiogenesis, and metastasis. Stopping angiogenesis (the development of new blood vessels) and the spread and metastasis of mutant cells is important to containing the growth of these damaged cells in the body.

It appears to do this in various cancer models by targeting several proteins in the mitochondrial signaling pathways. As you may recall, the mitochondria are the energy centers of cells. Hundreds of thousands of these structures surround a cell's nucleus, converting food energy into a form useful to that cell. Another function is to provide instructions in making the building blocks of amino acids, RNA, into functioning proteins, playing a role in signal pathways and regulatory events of cell growth. To sum it up, mitochondria are important to the body's biological balance.

With mitochondria signaling pathways playing a fundamental part in the proliferation of cells, as sensors of nutrients and physiological stress, blocking these pathways can play a central role in halting the spread and growth of mutated cancer cells. Laboratory research points to its ability to awaken genetic tumor suppression functions, contributing to the repair of damaged DNA or programming cell death, hence controlling and possibly stopping cancer increase before it can start.

Cinnamon

Cinnamon comes from the bark of the cinnamon tree. It is important to note that the research focuses on Ceylon cinnamon, sometimes called "real" cinnamon. This real cinnamon contains cinnamaldehyde, the bioactive compound that fights inflammation, and it also has properties that lower blood cholesterol and triglycerides. In lab testing, this essential oil assists in overcoming oxidative stress that can lead to cell damage and unchecked cancer.

From the pharmacological perspective, it seems most effective when used regularly, like any of these herbs and spices. I've found ways to include it in my daily diet by adding it to my coffee, tea, oatmeal, protein smoothies, sweet potatoes, on buttered toast with stevia or monk fruit sweetener, along with a myriad of other ways. I try to make it, along with other spices, a part of my regular intake of phyto-nutrients.

Holy Basil

Not to confuse it with sweet basil, used in many recipes for marinara sauce, nor with the Thai basil that adds much flavor to your favorite pho bowl, holy basil is considered a sacred herb in India, believed to help reach enlightenment, hence why it is called holy basil. It is substantive to Ayurvedic medicine, as far back as 1000 BC. Known botanically as tulsi or Ocimum sanctum linn, it promotes a healthy response to stress. The **National Library of Medicine** reports mounting evidence that tulsi helps contribute to various supportive aspects of your health through its unique pharmacological actions, exhibiting an ability to boost the immune system by encouraging the increase of the blood immune cells and cytokines.

Cytokines is an umbrella term for a diverse group of blood cells used to characterize proteins that carry molecular messages between cells, acting as immunoregulators. These proteins interact with immune system cells to balance the body's response to infections and disease. They are part of a complex process of cell physiology, interacting with immune cells to trigger a specific reaction, though are not limited to these actions.

Holy basil's seed oil extract's immunomodulatory effects show a statistical significance when compared to a placebo group. A supplemental 300 milligrams in capsule form of tulsi leaf extract, taken before food, was used for this study. There was a measurable increase in the levels of T-helper cells and NK-cells during this examination of the effectiveness of holy basil and cancer. T-cells are essential to regulating the immune response by modulating the activities of other immune cells and the behavior endothelial cells. One of the functions of the endothelial cells is to control the flow of white blood cells in and out of body tissue and through the vascular system.

NK cells, or natural killer cells, are best known for being aggressors towards viral infections and for detecting and attacking early signs of cancer; if you imagine a military tank, NK cells attack by shooting shells of the poison of perforin to create tiny openings like pores in the membranes of cancer cells, and releasing granzymes, which induces apoptosis in cancer cells, viruses, and bacteria, with the capacity to augment antibody and T-cell response, making them unique among the immune system cells. They play a pivotal role in protecting the body against cancers, acting as anti-cancer agents, swiftly killing cells that have transformed and begun the development of tumors.

The **National Institute of Health**'s account of five clinical studies reports that tulsi demonstrated an enhanced immune response. In a randomized study where neither the participants nor the experimenters knew which subjects were receiving what type of treatment, tulsi increased the number of NK cells and T-cells. This four-week investigation used 300mg of tulsi leaf extract daily without food, comparing healthy participants and placebo volunteers.

It is understandable why this "Queen of Herbs" has been a staple in the diet of many in India. The use of holy basil as an agent to enhance the immune system was known to ancient medical practitioners. It has been carried forward by some continuing the principles of these age-old methods. It appears that tulsi's leaf extract could contribute to today's cancer therapies as part of an integrative healthcare regimen.

Ginger

Ginger is well-known in the world of Asian cooking. It is one of those spices that adds a little punch to food. Many people enjoy the taste as it infuses just the right zest to a dish. You can also enjoy it as tea, sweetened with stevia or monk fruit and cooled, a healthy and refreshing drink.

Current research focuses on its two bioactive agents of gingerol and shogaol as the medicinal properties, both contained in the rhizome. Gingerol is a powerful anti-inflammatory and antioxidant and is possibly the most studied of the bioactive agents found in ginger. The

Yonsei Medical Journal, published by the **Yonsei University College of Medicine** in South Korea, conveyed some evidence that gingerol induces a stopping point of a pancreatic cancer cell's cycle so that it is no longer involved in duplication and division. The study was limited in scope, and more research is needed. Yet, it may be effective as a supplemental measure in your diet.

Another study, as disclosed by the **National Institute of Health**, discusses an investigation into the effects of ginger on many forms of cancer. One that stood out came after a review of 30 individuals who received 2 grams each day of gingerol extract. There was a significant reduction in pro-inflammatory signaling molecules in the colon, which is not surprising since ginger is touted as a useful digestive aid.

Cancer Prevention Research examined an investigation, in 2013, that followed 20 participants taking 2 grams of ginger or a placebo for 28 days. All the study's subjects were at high risk for colorectal cancer. Analysis of biopsies exhibited that ginger recipients had fewer negative changes in healthy colon tissue and diminished spread of corrupted unhealthy cells.

Shugaol, also an active agent that has also been studied in ginger, possessed significant inhibitory characteristics in reducing breast cancer cells and their spread in a controlled laboratory environment. Evidence indicates that shugaol impairs breast cancer cell invasion by targeting important pathways in cancer development and progression.

There is limited evidence that the compounds of gingerol and shugaol offer potential as effective natural agents against cancer. Whether you use ginger as an addition to your everyday diet, possibly as tea or in a meal, there is a benefit. Its major medicinal properties appear to be anti-inflammatory and antioxidant. Traditionally, ginger's use in helping with digestion and easing nausea may be helpful during chemo treatments. Incorporating ginger into your diet or as a supplement can support the body's efforts and lessen the unpleasantness you may experience from treatments.

Cumin

Cumin is a spice that comes from a plant that is from the parsley family. Its history as a spice goes back as far as 4000 years in the Middle East and is mentioned in both the Hebrew and Christian Testaments. It is commonly used in Mediterranean, Latin American, and Indian dishes, and frequently in American recipes of chili. While used for its intense flavor in cooking and roasting, cumin's essential oil offers many potential benefits.

The phytochemicals in seed spices offer high levels of beneficial bioactive compounds, and cumin is in that group. With its ability to impact various cellular systems, cumin genuinely influences health. Research shows promising benefits from using its essential oil in protecting the body from multiple forms of cancer.

Most of the investigation into cumin and its medicinal value has centered around the oil from black cumin, nigella sativa, offering a safe and promising anti-cancer agent. Records from some studies indicate a significant decrease in the incidence of both abnormal growth of tissue and liver cancer cells and the ability to inhibit the introduction of gastric squamous cell carcinoma, a scarce form of gastric malignancy. In lab studies, the **Journal of Nutrition and Cancer** noted a significant shrinking in size or slowing of the rate of tumorigensis in the stomach.

Thymoquinone (TQ), the most abundant and essential oil component from black cumin seeds, is a phytochemical compound known as anti-inflammatory, antioxidant, and antimicrobial, and has exhibited liver protective properties. Its chemopreventative abilities and promoting corrective action against chemically induced carcinogenesis support the investigation of an emerging compound as an anti-cancer chemical.

When reviewing the effects of TQ, possibly the most noted transformation was the increase of glutathione, one of the body's natural detoxifiers. Though its role is multifunctional, this agent of glutathione reacts with damaging environmental chemicals and free radicals to form harmless, inactive products for excretion from the body.

There is also considerable evidence that indicates the capacity of TQ to contain cancer cell proliferation in some diseases, including breast adenocarcinoma, ovarian carcinoma, bone cell cancer, pancreatic carcinoma, and one I'm familiar with, acute myeloblastic leukemia. The immunomodulatory effects of this agent warrant justification for including it as a dietary supplement to boost the immune system.

The findings of the pharmacological activities found in cumin and its application in traditional medicines of healing compounds of TQ and cumin aldehyde are now under investigation by science. They may become a part of a drug or drugs in the next generation of chemotherapy. When it comes to cancer prevention, protection from reoccurrence, enhancement to treatments, and recovery, cumin's essential oil is an important form of spice worth consideration.

Cloves

As a young Cub Scout, I still recall taking Styrofoam balls and filling them with whole cloves and sticking them all over the outside to form a fragrant ornament to hang on our Christmas tree. Today, around Thanksgiving and through the holiday season, I love the smell of a combination of apple, cinnamon, and cloves that fills the air when warmed in a pot on the stove or released from a diffuser. Did you know cloves contain effective compounds considered anti-cancer agents?

Appearing in a paper written on oncology research, cloves contain eugenol, a compound that is more effective at stopping oxidative damage than vitamin E. In lab testing of ethyl acetate (EAEC), a bioactive compound in cloves, it has revealed to scientists that it stimulates anti-tumor activities, including inhibitory characteristics, when applied to human colon cancer, breast, cervical, liver, and pancreatic cancer.

In the laboratory testing with Xenografts, when tissue from one species is transplanted to another, EAEC demonstrated the ability to significantly suppress the growth of cancer cells when compared to a control group. Also observed during this research was the apoptosis of malignant cells. The **International Journal of Applied Research in Oncology** reports a synergistic effect may be possible in combining EAEC with 5-fluorouracil-based chemotherapy.

It seems this cell death activity increased with longer exposure to EAEC. These occurrences were through the upregulation of cyclin-dependent kinase or CDK; cyclins are a family of proteins that control the progression of cells through the cell cycle. These CDKs inhibitors impede enzymes from acting as catalysts by regulating the RNA transcription, messengers of genetic material, needed to transfer DNA information required for the expression of genes.

All the results have been limited to laboratory testing, and human trials are necessary to evaluate its effectiveness. Yet, EAEC presents the possibility of an additional novel approach to using therapeutic herbs and spices for cancer. Finding a way to include cloves in your diet may favor keeping mutated cells at bay. Add cloves to your green tea, fruit salads, soups, and other creative possibilities. Using cloves as a daily routine may not cure cancer, but it could augment conventional care and become an essential step in prevention.

Studies have shown that some spices and herbal supplements are safe and effective. However, some have big claims attached to them, and their effectiveness has not been tested or shown to be possibly harmful or toxic to you. This material is only for educational purposes and is intended as information to be included with conventional therapies, not as a substitute. It is important to keep your caregiver informed anytime you choose to include these spices and herbs in your daily practices.

Including spices and herbs in building a winning approach amidst your crusade against cancer can be a valuable resource. Increasing recognition of the integrative concept of health is progressively recognized as one of the most effective ways to deal with any chronic disease. Your diet must develop into a synergistic part of a long-term path to better well-being. To expect positive results without decisive and affirmative actions, is folly. Now is a good time to do your part.

Chapter 9

I Owe, I Owe, Back to Work I Go, Not!

"Quit worrying about your health. It'll go away."
– Robert Orben

My initial bone marrow stem-cell transplant was autologous—harvesting my own—then implanted back into my body, which took place in January of 2010. I followed the guidance of eating more fruits and vegetables. I was working part time at various jobs and had plenty of energy. With over a year under my belt since my transplant, I felt incredible, so it was time to return to what I love—flying.

As I discussed earlier, a pilot must maintain a medical certificate to exercise the privileges of their license. Without that medical, it is as if they are not a licensed pilot. I enlisted the help of Dr. Cowl of the Mayo Clinic's Aero Medical division to jump through all the government's hoops to regain my medical certification. This occupational division at the Mayo Clinic cooperates with the military services, NASA, and the FAA, setting and maintaining requirements for healthy pilots.

In the late summer of 2011, I began to wake in the middle of the night with my t-shirt damp. I'd been there before, during stressful periods, so why was I stressed? Was it related to returning to flying? As the nights passed, the dampness increased to include my pajama bottoms, resulting in changing clothing in the middle of the night.

It wasn't long before running three days a week became a more significant challenge. Soon, climbing the stairs in our house ended with me pausing to catch my breath. Along with these new dilemmas, my night sweats resulted in changing clothing twice and, on occasion, three times each night. Hint, hint.

If that wasn't enough to get me to pay attention, waking one morning in December with a bloody nose spurred me to take action. On my way to the dentist for a cavity, I called my local oncologist, Dr. Brennen, and described the experiences of the last few months. He was emphatic in his answer: "You need to come in and see me." I canceled the dental appointment and drove directly to his office.

Upon arrival, the staff drew my blood. The results were that I was anemic; I had a low number of red blood cells carrying oxygen, and lacked palettes, cells involved in the clotting process. So, after an initial consultation, I was going to be admitted to the hospital for a much-needed blood transfusion and observation. But first, I had to call my wife Beth with the news.

I stepped outside and, with incredible resolve to not distress her, I made the call. Then, I took a breath and began disclosing the news of the current predicament. As I did, my emotions got the better of me and I began to cry. I felt like I had lost my battle. She immediately left work and came to the hospital to be beside me.

After staying overnight in the hospital, Dr. Brennan released me to go home, with instructions to return every few days for observation, blood draws, and transfusions when necessary. During this time, I received the diagnosis of pre-leukemia, or myelodysplastic syndrome (MDS). This period was incredibly emotionally challenging for me. Recall my father's story and how he passed; MDS was the beginning of the final months of his life. It was difficult for me to surrender those memories. But I had to, so that I could stay focused on my efforts to be a victor.

Recall the story of the Titanic and its sinking: With one section of the hull compromised by damage from an iceberg, water could flood through the whole ship because there were no barriers in the framework to prevent it. From this event, shipbuilders learned the importance of sectioning a ship into compartments, to insulate impaired chambers to protect the rest of the vessel. I prepared by putting this aspect of my life into a "day-tight compartment," a term coined by Sir William Osler, a physician and a founder of John Hopkins Hospital, focusing my efforts on the current challenge. With my active mind, this is not easy.

Doctor Brennan again went to bat for me and arranged a consultation at the Mayo Clinic. I met Dr. Mark Litzow, from the hematology department, and a professor at their prestigious medical school. He explained the blood disorder as acute myeloid leukemia (AML), and sadly, the chemotherapy used to rid me of multiple myeloma corrupted my bone marrow cells, compromising their genetic makeup.

Unfortunately, this can occur in a small percentage of people who receive this form of treatment. (Lucky, I am). Therefore, there was the need for a new bone marrow stem cell transplant from an outside donor. From our meeting came a treatment plan, and the beginning of the search for a donor. I started with my brothers and sisters and was fortunate that I had two brothers, Rick and Mike, that were perfect matches.

After receiving the plan from Dr. Litzow, I returned home to meet with Dr. Brennan to discuss starting treatments. With the Christmas holidays on the horizon, he was agreeable to me spending them with my family before beginning the arduous chemotherapy journey of 24 hours a day for seven days. I checked into the hospital on the 27th of December for a week of pure pampering of cocktails of daunorubicin and cytarabine. The purpose was to wipe out the leukemia cells and prepare for the regimen that would remove the existence of my bone marrow in readiness to introduce my brother's healthy cells. Let's get this party started.

From the bloody nose to the meeting with Dr. Litzow, a mind shift from fear to determination took place as I compartmentalized my focus to doing whatever it took not to be a victim of the disease. If I had a limited amount of time, I would live in the present as I prepare for an unknown future. I increased my efforts to eat healthier by adding more vegetables and related smoothies, while spending time in prayer/meditation, admittedly because of fear and not knowing what else I could do to strengthen my peace of mind.

The hospital staff was incredible and accommodating. During the day, visitors came by, and medical caregivers stopped in to answer questions and inform me what I could expect in the coming days and weeks. Late at night, I would roam the hallways, chemo tower in tow, in an effort to continue to be active and as a stress release so I might sleep better. The seven days passed relatively quickly, and I was released from the hospital to return home.

With my immune system highly compromised, I was susceptible to foreign pathogens from the outside world—and a hospital is full of them—and those that may already exist within my own body. Every day, I traveled to the oncology department in the hospital for outpatient care, monitoring, and as-needed blood transfusions. During one of these visits, my temperature began to rise during a transfusion. When this occurs, all actions stop or slow to give the host's body, which would be me, a period of adjustment. When the process began again, upward climbed my temperature. So, I received instructions to go home to rest and return the next day.

While lying in bed at home, I began to feel very chilled. Beth brought me more blankets while prompting me to go to the emergency room. I fought her on taking anything to control my fever or returning to the hospital. It wasn't until I was shivering uncontrollably, and she took my temperature, which read 104.4 degrees Fahrenheit, that I relented and went to the hospital.

Because of my condition, I was quickly admitted, and a series of tests took place to determine the seriousness of my situation. It took a while for the results to return, but the staff continuously brought me warm blankets to help with the shivering that didn't seem to stop, even after being given medicine to help control the fever. The test results were definitive—I had pneumonia.

I lay in the emergency room bed for hours while the search for a suitable room began. I needed a private room, thoroughly disinfected, because my immune system was compromised. Finally, later in the evening, I was transferred to my new resident bed to experience the scariest and most threatening part of the cancer journey.

As the hours grew into the next day, my conversations became very difficult. I needed to take a series of breaths in mid-sentence. My oxygen levels had dropped below 88 percent, so I began supplemental oxygen. My communication ability grew worse, as I could only say a few words before the need to "catch my breath." Dr. Brennan once told me that many cancer patients die of other complications and not from the disease. This came to the forefront of my mind.

During my trial with pneumonia, an infectious disease doctor came to visit me. He ordered new chest X-rays to be taken of the lungs to see if the pneumonia was progressively getting worse. The X-ray results indicated that it had indeed worsened, and the need to determine just what kind and possibly its origin. An operation was scheduled to biopsy my lungs to determine what was growing there, and to decide on an effective treatment.

The biopsy taken from the lungs identified strep mitis bacteremia as the cause of pneumonia. So, intravenous antibiotics were introduced to me through the chemotherapy port in my chest. But what was of significant interest to the doctors was that these bacteria are typically in the digestive tract. The question was, how did it get up into my lungs?

Here is where ignorance and asking dumb questions can open the doors of possibilities. I asked if these bacteria could originate in the mouth? He acknowledged that it was possible. Returning to the morning of the bloody nose, weeks earlier, and how I was supposed to see the dentist to care for a cavity, I thought there might be a connection. The infectious disease physician believed that there was a possibility. But, for now, I had to get healthy.

After a continuous flow of antibiotics and my immune system rebuilding itself from the hammering it took from earlier chemotherapy, I was beating pneumonia. Finally, after more than seven days into my hospital stay, I could have the oxygen removed as my oxygen levels were 97 percent. Three days later, I was released and returned home.

Within a few days of arriving home, I received a phone call from Dr. Litzow, explaining that from his review of the test results after the chemotherapy, he believed I would benefit from another round of the delightful chemo-cocktail I partook in December and January. Of course, with the most recent pneumonia experience fresh in my mind, I was not excited about the possibility of a repeat on the road just taken. But with great respect for him and his background, I was willing and able to go another bout with this AML opponent. But, first, I had that darn cavity repaired, before I took another go at preparing for my defeat of this adversary.

Round two was the same as the first, except for no other complications like pneumonia. Again, I felt good, other than fatigue, most of the time following the same outpatient protocols as the original. After a few weeks of recovery, I left for the Mayo Clinic with my donor brother, Mike, as an escort.

Over a smattering of days in Rochester, Minnesota, Mike attended several appointments, including meeting with a counselor, who had the unfortunate task of explaining what I was already aware of: In the worst-case scenario, his cells may detect my own body as an adversary, and attack them, resulting in the possibility of my demise. That idea shook him to the core. But with further explanation, even with that as a threat, he understood that he was my best chance at living and being around for my family—and, of course, to harass him, as is the job of an older brother.

When it came time for Mike to donate his bone marrow stem cells, he was an overachiever. What took me four days to accomplish when they took my stem cells for my autologous transplant, he did in one day. Show off. He came, he conquered, but he didn't get a t-shirt; just some aches from his body manufacturing so many stem cells—some for me and some for him.

Just before Easter, Mike flew home, and I checked into the hospital for observation until Beth came for the transplant. Before that, another round of chemo was in store for me to kill my remaining bone marrow and make way for my brother's healthy stem cells. You never get used to that stuff, but I am fortunate to tolerate chemotherapy with only little discomfort. Next up was transplant day.

On March 29, 2012, a day that within our family has come to be known as my rebirth day, is one I share with my son Joseph's actual birthday, Beth accompanied me to the Mayo Clinic to meet my new "little friends," my brother's stem cells. The stem cells were administered through an IV into the port in my chest. As I had been through this before with my stem cells and it was uneventful, I suggested to Beth, if she'd like, to go somewhere for lunch or shop, because this takes four or more hours, and I was in the excellent care of the nursing staff and doctors.

Everything was going well until it wasn't. Different from when I received my stem cells, these were foreign to my body and it let me know that it was not happy, by raising my temperature, making me feel nauseous, and having my bowls decide to purge themselves. Recall that the gut is an essential part of the immune system, so it was doing its job of fighting invaders. Or maybe, my brother was getting revenge on me for all the teasing I did to him through the years growing up.

During this period, Beth returned to find I was in some distress. I got out of bed and rolled my IV tree, with stem cells in tow, to the bathroom before everything let loose in the bed. While I was switching between kneeling before the porcelain god and sitting on the throne, Beth had alerted the staff to my predicament.

A knock on the bathroom door came, asking how I was doing. "Not so good!" was my response. I explained my situation. Through the door came this cute young nurse, grabbing the trash can for me to barf into, if necessary, to assist as I sat in all my glory. A sudden shift to embarrassment came over me. It wasn't exactly the position a man wants to be in around a young lady. Her professionalism overcame my humiliation as she tended to me.

She stopped the stem cells flow from the IV bag, allowing my body to adjust to these new immigrants. After a while, my body adapted to these strangers and I began to feel less discomfort. I soon made it back to my bed and rested awhile before trying again. When the nurse restarted the IV, this time the drip was more gradual, enabling my body to accommodate these regenerative and hopefully prolific new companions.

The rest of the transplant took place without any complications. It was time to hope and pray that these healthy cells would feel at home within my body and become fruitful and multiply. In 3 to 4 days, a blood test indicated an increase in various cells. After the implanted stem cells settled in, they would produce new ones, becoming any cell needed by the body. Some days my white blood cells increased, while other times, it might be the red blood cells surging forward in numbers or platelets. I needed all of them.

During the months following my transplant, a steady flow of caregivers, my sisters, brothers, and friends, including my mother-in-law, came to watch over me while living in Rochester at The Transplant House, a place dedicated to—you guessed it—transplant patients. Here we were, sharing a living space with a group of people from very diverse backgrounds worldwide, everyone with a common goal—to be healthy—becoming friendly with many, sitting in rocking chairs enjoying a sunny day while conversing or listening to music, with someone playing guitars and banjos, and sharing traditional meals from each other's cultures, victories, and defeats. It was a very positive and enjoyable experience; it wasn't home, but it made it more bearable.

The days usually began with appointments at the clinic, before being free for the afternoons. Fortunately, spring came early, so we took advantage it, walking or riding bikes on the incredible trail system they have in and around the city. My progress continued with an occasional blip on the radar but no major setback. When in discussion with Dr. Litzow about one of those issues, I queried him about whether or not

I should be less active or change my diet, His response was to keep doing what I was doing because it was working. I credit much of this to having a perfectly matched donor, and also to the habits I developed in life, especially my dietary shift after my initial diagnosis of multiple myeloma. Because things continued in a positive manner, my release from Mayo came in June instead of the expected month of July.

Once I returned home, there were weekly follow-up appointments, with once-a-month IV therapy that was to enhance the possibility of survival. I met people who were fighting their own battles with various forms of cancer, each with a unique story to tell. One woman I met, lost her struggle, but in our conversations, I sensed she was not a victim. I was impressed with her positive attitude, how she lived in the present, and her willingness to not let cancer steal her spirit.

In April 2013, with the help of Dr. Cowl at the Mayo Clinic, I was permitted to return to flying. The FAA medical administrator gave me a special issuance, with some strict guidelines that had to be met so that I could maintain my medical qualifications, including regular blood samples and a letter from Dr. Litzow pertaining to my health. The head medical examiner for the FAA, personally advised me that it was a first, but with input from Dr. Cowl, she believed I was a good candidate to receive this special issuance. I am happy to say that after 10 years of continued good health, I have been released from those strict requirements.

Thankfully, Mike's stems cells, implanted in me, continue to be just as enthusiastic to give me a longer life as they were when first donated. Thanks, bro.

Chapter 10

And Another Thing

"Better to light a candle than curse the darkness."
– Chinese Proverb

If you're like me and are constantly interested in learning new things, you may be familiar with epigenetics. If you aren't, it's not surprising since it is still in its infancy. So, very quickly, epi is Greek for "above" or "in addition." Think of epigenetics as altering a gene's genetic expression or function without a change or mutation. Our genes don't change, but their behaviors do, as our lifestyle, diet, and physical habits influence them. Research in epigenetics investigates what and how genes are expressed as a normal part of bodily function. These studies have changed the understanding of what leads to chronic diseases like cancer and autoimmune diseases. According to Bruce Lipton, a microbiologist and author of the book *Biology of Belief*, in the past, the belief was that your genes were responsible for up to 70 percent of the destiny of your health. If your parents had a chronic disease, you had a 70 percent chance you would also experience the same chronic illness. Now the belief is that this is not necessarily so.

Science has begun to shift thinking as to health and genotype. In contrast, diseases may be more of a result from one's environment, including lifestyle, traumatic experiences, stress, toxins, infections and disease, drugs and medications, dietary habits, amount and quality of regular exercise, and lack of proper rest. These are influencers of genetic expression or phenotype. A phenotype is how your body expresses your genetic makeup.

But when the immune response is in disarray, one may experience autoimmune diseases like rheumatoid arthritis, allergies, chronic inflammation, and cancer. Food is an important component in creating balance and is an influencer of the immune system and possibly genetic expression. It's one of the primary ways the outer world interacts with the human body's complex networks, especially the immune system. The best prescription for a more positive phenotypic adaptation is to create an environment in the body and mind that promotes a balanced immune response.

A misconception about cancer is that treatments only delay the inevitable. But I refused to accept that the patient cannot do anything to affect a better outcome. What we do in life matters. One sphere of influence you can affect starting today is your health. There are practical steps an individual can take that can act as personal medicines to supplement what the medical community is doing on your behalf.

These antidotes range from improving your diet, reducing stress, getting regular exercise, and having a more positive approach towards the journey and all of life's experiences. Implementing changes in these areas can power up the body's natural defenses to fight cancer better and aid it in the recovery process. Winning the battle is a multifaceted process in which you must actively participate. The sooner, the better the results. But you have to get started, so don't wait. Even if you don't have cancer or any other chronic disease, you can benefit from improving these areas. Your actions, or lack of activities, make a difference.

We need the motivation to change our lives. If you played sports, did well in school, played a musical instrument, or pursued a dream or goal to fulfillment, there was some driving influence that kept you going when you didn't feel like it. Most things that get done in this world are by people who, at some point, have questioned whether or not it's worth it. They had a motivator, a purpose to help them focus on the desired outcome.

To win over cancer, you will need reasons to engage in the battle to realize the best possible outcome, whatever you define that to be. What are you passionate about that will empower you to believe it is all worthwhile? That is an individual decision, and only you can answer that question. Before anything changes, you must decide, "I ain't gonna live like this anymore." Then get started being the physically and mentally healthy person you desire to be. One step, one step, one step... Oops, I moved backward a couple of squares. It happens. Now start from where you are and keep moving positively forward. You can do it.

You must have a big enough **WHY** to push you forward after the news of an unexpected setback—a strong desire to not quit when test results are not the good news hoped for. For example, when you feel tired and miserable, you must force yourself to eat nutritious foods when every bite tastes like a chemical because of chemo. But you eat it, even though it may lead to nausea and knowing you may kneel before the porcelain throne soon.

I knew a woman who beat the doctor's timeline after being diagnosed with pancreatic cancer. She was able to be a part of her daughter's wedding, helping her plan it, select a dress, and participate as a co-presenter—along with her husband—of the bride's hand to the groom. She also was able to see the face of her newborn grandchild before her life came to an end. That was her victory over cancer. What's yours?

We all need something bigger than us alone. Achievement of great things comes to realization when purpose drives us. If you haven't already, take some time to determine a reason to stand up and challenge this condition that has hijacked your body and life. See it, know it, and mostly feel the **WHY** of winning. Once you know what inspires you, that may be all it takes to empower you to do whatever is needed, to find a new, more confident you.

Personally, when I was diagnosed with my second cancer, what concerned me the most was leaving my wife behind to raise three young boys under the age of ten. Add to it a business deal I was responsible for getting us into, which had gone bad. We sold many assets to cover the debt and had to refinance our house to keep us out of bankruptcy. Contemplating some negative scenarios would bring tears to my eyes. Being there for my family physically, emotionally, and financially became my driving force.

Thanks to some great friends and family members who planned, organized, and spread the word to former schoolmates and others through conversations, an amazing fundraiser for my medical bills took place. I am forever grateful to those who gave so much time and effort, donated, and came together that evening. It enabled us to cover all the cancer-related bills.

I challenge you with this intimate question that you must answer from your heart: "Do you want to win?" More potently, "Why must you win?" The answers to these questions may be the driving energy that pushes you to do whatever it takes to release the grip of cancer. An empowering purpose provides an unwavering determination to win.

Time matters. Don't delay. Decide today that you are ready to take on this formidable foe. Develop an attitude of, **"I may have cancer, but I will not let the cancer get me."** Even if you succumb to the disease, do your best not to give in to it and allow it to take whatever joy you can find in each new day and in the people around you. Become an example for others, to live with courage. It will change the rest of your life and may positively change others watching. When I asked the disempowering question, "Why me?" I believe I received a divinely inspired answer: "To demonstrate courage for others." A response from my creator or not, it was empowering, and I decided, "To be, it was up to me."

If you only accept things as they are, you are unlikely to develop a possibility attitude that accompanies a winning mindset. Reasonable people accept what is, without challenging it. While unreasonable people see what is, focus on where they want to go, and do the irrational anyway. Be unreasonable. Having determination to do whatever and everything it takes, then acting on it with a spirit of living, is what it takes to get through it. If your attitude is "fix me, doc,"

I believe you will be gravely disappointed. If it's more like, "What can I do to help the doctors succeed?" greater possibilities exist.

Do not accept everything a doctor says as the only possibility. There may be additional options, such as an integrative practitioner. Visit the **Mayo Clinic's** integrative medicine department and explore new possibilities. There are many possible avenues one can travel when dealing with a disease. Common in Western societies and conventional for cancer include radiation and chemotherapy. Both are effective. Along with these treatments, consider additional options to have in your regiments like natural medicines. These therapies are in addition to or complementary to conventional medicine.

Ayurvedic (a-yer-va-dik) means the science of life and has its historical roots in the Indian subcontinent. It is a system of holistic health practices involving the mind, body, and spirit, encompassing lifestyle, diet, and exercise. It's an individual complementary approach to health.

The Western alternative could be homeopathic medicine that embraces a holistic and natural way of treating an illness. Like Ayurvedic, it focuses on the whole person, not just on a disease. Rooted in the traditions of the father of Greek medicine, Hippocrates, it is totality in method and not disease specific. It comprises the physical, psychological, and emotional characteristics of the patient.

Some medical providers trained at modern medical schools will shoot these ideas down as "quackery," but it should be up to you to decide whether they are helpful. Some have a basis in scientific thinking but not necessarily in a lab or systematic testing. Learn as much as possible through your research to make an informed decision. Be sure to choose from a reliable information provider, such as NIH library, Cleveland Clinic, or available Mayo Clinic publications.

Winning is a process. Some people refuse to accept a final word as the closing chapter of an incomplete story. It is up to you to create your epic journey by living as fully and capably as possible. It may be the closing chapter of a life fulfilled or setting the stage for the sequel to your new story. Either way, do your best to find as much joy each day, each moment.

Organic or Not, That is the Question

As intelligent as you are (I know because you're reading this book), it is obvious to you that eating between five and ten fruits and vegetables a day is necessary for quality health. Additionally, there is value in consuming produce grown organically over those cultivated with conventional agricultural practices. Everyday farming uses pesticides, and mounting evidence identifies exposure to these chemicals with an increase in chronic diseases like neurodegenerative ones, cancer, and others, with agricultural workers being the most at risk.

Organics can be much more expensive than conventionally grown fruits and vegetables. Possibly start with eating naturally grown foods that typically aren't peeled, such as berries, fruits like apples and peaches, spinach, and other leafy greens. The least contaminated are usually melons, avocados, mushrooms, cabbage, and asparagus, to name a few, along with some others.

The EPA website states, "...The health effects of pesticides depend on the type of pesticide." And, "Some pesticides may be carcinogens. Others may affect the hormone or endocrine system in the body." The **Frontiers in Public Health**, self-described as an "...open-access journal which publishes rigorously peer-reviewed research..." identifies a possible risk by, "The combination of substances with probably carcinogenic or endocrine-disrupting effects may produce unknown adverse health effects. Therefore, the determination of "safe" levels of exposure to single pesticides may underestimate the real health effects, ignoring also the chronic exposure to multiple chemical substances."

By some standards, European regulation of pesticides may be the most restrictive on Earth. Information appearing in **Research Gate**, a website for sharing science-related information, offers that "...experts in toxicology, law, and policy, identified shortcomings in the authorization process..." Also, "...a growing body of evidence shows that pesticides that have passed through this process and are authorized for use may harm humans, animals, and the environment." It may be time to reevaluate how governments determine the safety of such products since the information regulatory agencies rely on, as provided by the manufacturer, may be biased.

An assessment of apples noted a higher concentration of residual chemicals, exceeding acceptable toxicology standards, presenting a possible health hazard, especially for children. By eating organically grown foods, it may be possible to decrease the amount of residual pesticide exposure. Unless you plant and raise fruits and vegetables in a personal garden, it is unlikely that they are chemically free, since many organic farmers will use some insect or weed control approved by the EPA as organic in origin.

After reviewing separate studies on the effects of organic and conventional foods, researchers from **Stanford University** determined eating organics did not necessarily provide any more nutritional value. Yet, organics do offer lower exposure to harmful chemicals, and analysis of the information available is murky as to how long-term exposure to pesticides from food may affect health. If organics are too costly, do not allow that to stop you from reaping the rewards of the vital and valuable nutrients available in fruits and vegetables—eating conventionally grown produce is far better than eating limited amounts or none.

Regardless of the source, washing them before eating or during preparation is valuable. There are commercially available rinses, but research indicates that rinsing under cold running water is as effective as most store-bought cleaners. A study published in the **JOURNAL of AGRICULTURAL and FOOD CHEMISTRY** found that a home alternative of soaking produce in a weak solution of 1-ounce baking soda to 100 ounces of water for approximately 15 minutes, followed by a cold-water rinse, was the most effective way to remove these chemicals from your fruits and vegetables. It is crucial to dry them afterward to prevent mold and reduce the probability of bacteria growing. Adding a paper towel to the storage container seems to reduce moisture problems and help prolong its freshness.

Lifestyle

How we live—our behaviors, attitudes, food, and drink; pretty much whatever we do or not do that influences a way of life—equates to lifestyle. According to epigenetic researchers, it is one area that impacts genetic expression. To become a victor over cancer, decide to do all you can do, and your lifestyle is something you control regardless of disease, treatments, or doctors' personal bias. It's simple and takes nothing more than the willingness to make a shift, and the support of those who will take the journey with you.

Exercise

The health and wellness community says that a sedentary lifestyle is the new smoking, and we know how unhealthy that is. Exercise and a positive mental attitude are vital foundations for a healthy lifestyle. Though regularly working out and doing aerobic exercises may not prevent a disease like cancer, research cataloged by **the US National Library of Medicine** shows it can help control and prevent disease.

Any of us can agree that exercising increases one's ability to perform physically; this is called performance status. Moreover, according to **Current Treatments Options in Oncology**, it may be a valuable predictor of a patient's chances of surviving many types of cancer. Exercises that work both the heart and lungs are aerobic. They considerably improve our performance status. It reduces related problems arising from treatments while allowing you to get the most from them.

Dr. James Turner and Dr. John Campbell, distinguished physiologists from **University of Bath's Department for Health,** site a benchmark study from 2018, saying exercise boosts the immune system's ability to handle pathogens. Over the long run, it decreases changes to the immune system that occur as we age, lowering the dangers of infections.

An article in **Medicine & Science in Sports & Exercise**, a monthly peer-review journal, documents that exercise counters internal inflammation, a driver of chronic diseases like cancer, by promoting the development of anti-inflammatory molecules while also stimulating an increase of macrophage, a type of white blood cell that act as scavengers circulating through the blood and hanging out in the liver and lymph nodes, looking for and trapping foreign microbes to ingest like a tiny Pac-Man.

Evidence supports including a program of physical activities as a part of a cancer treatment plan. Appearing in **Harvard Health Publishing**, a circulation of evidence-based and trustworthy information, Dr. Prue Cormie of the **Clinical Oncology Society of Australia (COSA)** states, "If we could turn the benefits of exercise into a pill, it would be demanded by patients, prescribed by every cancer specialist, and then subsidized by the government. It would be seen as a major breakthrough in cancer treatment."

Monique Tello, MD, writes in the same **Harvard Medical School** publication, "There are hundreds of studies showing real, tangible benefits of exercise for patients with various cancers and at different stages. Exercise specifically as an additional therapy for cancer patients has been well-studied and associated with many benefits."

An analysis of trials involving more than 1000 people with cancers such as lung, multiple myeloma, lymphoma, and others, varying in stages from I to IV, and comparing those who followed exercise guidelines to those who did not, showed that the exercising participants had more energy, greater strength, a better quality of life, and experienced less anxiety and depression. They also enjoyed improved health-related outcomes.

A **Mayo Clinic** article stated, "Research confirms that exercising can help you not just survive but thrive during and after cancer." Shara Mansfield, a certified cancer exercise trainer at **Mayo Clinic Healthy Living Program**, says too much rest "can lead to functional decline. Research tells us, in general, it's better to move more than less." But will it assist in winning the fight against cancer? Again, from the **Mayo Clinic**, "Studies have found that exercise during treatment can actually change the tumor microenvironment and trigger stronger anti-tumor activity in your immune system." In addition, recent laboratory experiments have established that regular exercise leads to a reduction in tumor size.

Exercise helps the lymph system to flush impurities from the body. Unlike the circulatory system, which has the heart as its pump, there isn't one for the lymph system. Instead, it relies on the movement of muscles to pump fluid through them, remove contaminants, and eliminate them as part of the body's natural cleansing.

Consistent physical activity is essential to health. Your actions can be as simple as bicycling a few times a week, walking for 20 to 30 minutes daily, working out at a gym, or even playing golf. That means walking the course, not riding in a cart with a cooler full of beer; that's a social benefit. Focus on moderate-vigorous, aerobic-type activities, with a target of approximately three hours each week as all that is needed to achieve healthful benefits. Keep it simple, desirable and easy to do.

Walking is a perfect example. It can become a social event when you include others and conversation. Or when you go shopping, park further away to increase the distance to an entrance. If shopping involves a mall, go early and walk around before shopping. Making it as brisk as possible is one the best ways to stay agile, keeping the joints loose and allowing the blood to flow, therefore getting food and medicine where needed. Challenge yourself to walk stairs instead of taking an elevator, if able. Adopt new hobbies like dancing and gardening.

Strength-building exercises can range from weight training to resistance bands; Pilates and yoga are mind-body exercises and can be an excellent way to relax and release stress, as is tai chi, which is a slow and deliberate form of martial arts—just about anything you can think of that makes you try harder by pushing, pulling, or holding a distinct position. For example, planks or sitting with your back against a wall without a chair, or whatever challenges your muscles to do more than the daily motions of life. The function of the immune system intensifies with the increase of lean muscle mass due to resistance training. Additional benefits include improved skeletal muscle strength and bone density and enhanced neurological responses, to cite a few.

In addition to maintaining muscle strength, yoga and Pilates benefit the gut. The bending and twisting motions help move food through your digestive tract and release stress. A **Sports Medicine** review indicates that gentle movement of a moderate pace exercise appears more favorable to the gut than vigorous, more aggressive forms of training. A healthy gut biome with proper flora is necessary to get the most out of your foods, especially during this time of maximum nutritional needs.

Ask for recommendations for training practitioners from your health professional. If they can't or aren't willing to provide you with a referral, look to the American College of Sports Medicine for certified trainers who specialize in working with people undergoing cancer treatment and those who want to continue to thrive after their diagnosis. Whomever you choose, be sure they are accredited and familiar with the area of fitness as it pertains to cancer care.

The form of physical activity you choose is not as important as it is to keep moving. If you already have a routine, don't stop. Just be sure to consult with your physician to verify it fits your therapy phase. Your fitness level, treatment stage, and the chronic condition you have determines your intensity of effort. The aim is moderate intensity, but the magnitude of exertion is to align with your physical condition and abilities. Avoid strenuous exercise because your body needs its storehouse of energy to repair and regenerate damaged tissue during treatments. A little exercise beats none while still allowing for the body's need to mend as your strength returns. Increase your frequency or try greater exertion to challenge the body. But keep it reasonable. It's not about getting ripped or looking gorgeous in a bikini; that comes later.

The cancer diagnosis taught me that being in shape does not transfer to being healthy. Healthy living influences a healthy body, with exercise as an essential contribution but not the only part.

Sleep

Good physical conditioning is a positive way to reduce feelings of anxiety and depression while increasing energy—something we all need, especially cancer patients. In addition, regular training can help you sleep better, improving your quality of life. A **Journal of Psychiatry and Neuroscience** report affirms that a daily activity routine encourages a positive mental outlook. When we are physically active, the brain's mood chemistry changes by releasing numerous neurotransmitters. Bodily exertion stimulates the release of endorphins, dopamine, norepinephrine, and serotonin. Each of these plays an essential role in a constructive and balanced mood.

Research on sleepiness demonstrates that it impairs judgment and our ability to assess situations in life effectively. Oddly enough, this includes how much sleep we need. Most of us in our youth thought we were functioning normally, despite our poor sleep habits. The experts say this is not so. Tests show that mental alertness is compromised; our performance and learning ability suffer. With continued lack of sleep, our effectiveness declines without us recognizing it. In the flying business, quality rest is essential for safe operations. If we aren't rested, we classify ourselves as unable to fly due to fatigue. You don't want a tired pilot responsible for your safety.

How well you sleep influences so many aspects of your life. According to the **Cleveland Clinic**, lack of valuable sleep can increase the chances of developing diabetes, depression and anxiety, cardiovascular diseases, and immune system impairment. Men, it can affect your sexual drive and performance. Ladies, it ages your appearance, making you look older because sleep deprivation increases cortisol, which breaks down skin collagen needed to keep the wrinkles at bay. Did I get your attention?

Rest is vital, and sleep is pivotal to enduring a cancer struggle. Quality and quantity of sleep are crucial to the rejuvenation of tissue and immunity cells. Components critical to healthy immune functions strengthen during the deepest stages of the sleep cycle. Interaction within the immune system helps it identify antigens it has dealt with, an immune memory known as acquired immunity. Once identified, it can then respond to the presence of an attacker. Sleep enables the body to slow other processes more dominant while awake, so that it can rev up the immune system to fight off foreign intruders. Restful slumber is vital in maintaining a robust immune system, enabling us to adapt to our environment successfully.

There appears to be a correlation between the abundance and variety of sleep and length of survival with some cancers. It shouldn't be surprising since lack of it is known to impair immunity against illnesses such as colds or the flu. Finally, we've all heard about the importance of "rest and recuperation" after an operation; a doctor at the Mayo Clinic once told me that chemotherapy is comparable to simultaneously operating on your whole body. So, rest and recuperation are critical to recovery.

The immune system generally mounts a defensive battle against intruders through a complex network. This organized design involves both inherited traits and acquired immunities. The inherited, also known as innate immunity, involves many defense tiers and allows the body to respond quickly to pathogens. In comparison, our acquired or adaptive immunity focuses on distinct threats and increases or grows over time, enabling us to live harmoniously with our environment, countering recognized unhealthy microorganisms. A sensitive balance between them is affected by the quality of sleep.

T-cells are an integral player in the immune community, a core component of the adaptive immune response. They are white blood cells acting as the body's special forces on search and destroy missions of a specific pathogen. A sticky protein called integrins is released when a T-cell recognizes an infected cell. The stickiness allows the T-cells to attach themselves to these cells, and even cancer cells, so that it can kill them. A challenge for integrins is that stress hormones reduce their ability to adhere to the bad players. Dr. Dimitrov, a German scientist studying sleep's effects on the immune system's functions, says his findings indicate that sleep can potentially improve T-cell effectiveness as stress hormones dip during the sleep cycle. Without this stickiness, these critical immune cells cannot perform effectively.

To the youthful citizens of the world, lack of sleep seems to be a way of life. I get it; I was there, staying late at parties and bars with friends, not fully functioning, according to science, the next day from exhaustion. Consistently sleeping less than five hours each night has been associated with a higher mortality rate. For many, seven hours is a typical night's sleep. But three nights in a row of less than seven hours, is the equivalent of one night without any rest. Get your zzz's; it is important to your overall health. Plus, you will feel and look better to others because your mood won't be ugly.

It's Supplemental

With an array of supplements on the market, the seller uses the premise of health-enhancing as a tactic of seduction. Through persuasion, vendors influence us to buy, convincing us they will enable us to be anyone from a male sexual dynamo to a superhuman. Many articles have some research behind the claims made by the marketing hype; some of the benefits are well known, while others seem to deserve no more than a "yeah right" exclamation. My email seems regularly filled with some blend of an ancient secret of the gods, that a mysterious stranger had to share before they passed on; otherwise, it will be lost to humankind forever.

Not to be a negative Ned; it's just an observation of the constant bombardment of the marketing tactics employed to play on our hopes and emotions that advertisers use to convince us to buy. Some of these products may contain only substances of limited value or possibly no advantage to your health. That is not to say that all supplements are useless. What I am saying is, if you are a consumer of various ones, as I am, they did not prevent you from getting cancer or any other chronic disease; so, by themselves, they are not likely to turn the tide on ill health.

Many people aren't aware that vitamins and supplements are not required to meet the same proof of effectiveness as drugs. Some sellers of these products make many generalized statements claiming miraculous results without qualifying evidence. The Federal Food and Drug Administration can pull a product off the market if it's proven dangerous. I have looked for research proving promising benefits in combating cancer.

Some supplements can be beneficial during treatments. For instance, I used aloe vera with vitamin E on my skin during radiation therapy to alleviate the pain from the burn caused by it, and it worked very effectively. In addition, vitamin C was recommended by my doctor to enhance my immune response while recovering from the first stem cell transplant regimen, along with an assortment of other vitamins I elected to use on my own. The following are some of the possible nourishing micronutrients that may be beneficial to enhancing cancer treatments and the body's natural response to it.

A valuable supplement is resveratrol, which shows some potential in enhancing cancer treatments, inducing apoptosis of cancer cells, and reducing the side effects of some therapeutics. Laboratory examinations indicate it has potential anti-cancer properties. My choice of resveratrol brand also includes a green tea extract of the catechins of EGCG, mentioned by Dr. Mark Hyman, a functional medicine practitioner, as "...some of the most powerful disease-fighting phytonutrients...." It also contains a grape seed extract of a bioflavonoid called proanthocyanidins. In lab testing, these compounds demonstrated anti-inflammatory properties and boosted the immune system by stimulating T-cell development and antioxidant potentially greater than vitamin C and E.

Supplements alone will not prevent you from getting cancer, or cure it. Eating an array of whole foods with their micronutrients is the most effective means of acquiring the vital compounds needed to beat cancer, yet diet alone may not be enough.

The recommended daily (dietary) allowance, or RDA, was established by the US Food and Nutrition Board as a guide for preventing malnutrition. But when battling cancer, the body may benefit from more than the minimum daily requirements. For example, in Japan, where fish is a primary protein source in their diet, a study involving fish oil supplements found that the survival rate among leukemia patients who received a bone marrow transplant was better than those who did not take fish oil.

The **JOURNAL of UROLOGY** referenced a study with bladder cancer patients that, in addition to the RDA, were given extra zinc, vitamins A, B6, C, and E, experienced a lower chance of reoccurrence than the group that did not supplement with these nutrients. The body's natural immune mechanisms may benefit from added vitamins and minerals or those missing in our diet. There are some instances when specific phytonutrients and vitamins work collaboratively with anti-cancer treatments for a more effective result.

As mentioned in both food and as a spice, garlic, or its active ingredient, allicin, is understood to be a powerful antioxidant. Laboratory testing, documented by the **National Cancer Institute**, indicates that allicin, along with other active compounds found in garlic, may lower the risk of some cancers. A **European Journal of Pharmacology** abstract expresses that "allicin inhibited the growth of cancer cells of murine and human origin." Also, "Antiproliferative effects of allicin partly account for the chemo-preventive action of garlic extracts...." Most studies of allicin use supplemental doses of 300 to 1500mg per day. It is necessary to mention that allicin extract can rapidly lose its medicinal value, and that in the previously cited lab testing, allicin was directly introduced to cancer cells. So, supplementation is good, yet garlic is most valuable when consumed regularly in a healthy diet.

The presence of vitamin D receptors in almost all immune cells points to their significant role in the healthy functioning of both innate and adaptive immune systems. Sunlight, foods with vitamin D, and supplementation with it can increase T-cell activity. Evidence continues to accumulate as to the negative consequences of vitamin D deficiency. A growing number of laboratory studies indicate vitamin D as a crucial part of the immune system. Along with its ability to act as a modulator of inflammation, it certainly makes having an ample quantity of it vital to our health.

Newer studies have found a correlation between a deficiency of vitamin D and some cancers, primarily those associated with the endocrine system or hormone-related, such as prostate and breast. The endocrine system functions much like the nervous system. But, instead of communicating with electrical impulses, it uses chemical transmitters called hormones to regulate various body functions. Sufficient levels of it may play a role in reducing the risk or preventing the reappearance of certain cancers. In laboratory studies, it was able to stop the uncontrolled growth of prostate cancer cell cultures, with similar results for colon and breast cancer cells.

The body naturally produces the "sun vitamin" with skin exposure to sunlight. The amount of time influences how much, along with where you live, northern regions versus southern, and increased sun time and the pigment of your skin; light skin produces up to five times as much vitamin D. The protective effects of melanin or darkness of the skin, require increased time in the sun to make the same amount of this vitamin. As a footnote, sunscreen provides valuable protection from ultraviolet damaging rays; it can also reduce vitamin D production.

Ongoing research suggests that a combination of calcium and vitamin D may act as a preventative to cancer, while insufficient levels could contribute to some types of cancer. While diet and sunlight are the best sources of vitamin D, supplements may be necessary, such as in winter months in some areas. The recommended daily allowance for vitamin D is between 400 international units (IU) for young children and up to 800 IU for people over 70. Over 4000 IU per day may be toxic.

A supplement that I take daily is coenzyme Q10 or CoQ10. It is essential for basic cell functions of growth and development and cell support. An antioxidant and anti-inflammatory produced naturally by the body, it helps to protect the heart and brain against certain cancers. Though the body can meet most CoQ10 requirements, with age comes a reduction in its capability to manufacture it. It is also present in certain foods such as nuts, eggs, and some cold-water fish like salmon and sardines, yet supplementation may be beneficial. Be sure to talk with your doctor, especially if you are on an anticoagulant medication such as warfarin.

Ginseng is a plant that covers 13 separate species. The most common forms of the supplement are Asian and American ginseng. Tests indicate ginseng acts as an anti-inflammatory, while red ginseng, whose color comes from its age, helps reduce oxidative stress.

Ginsenosides, one of the active agents in ginseng, have been shown in laboratory testing to decrease angiogenesis and metastasis of cancer cells and stimulate immune functions. It is also described as having various other healing characteristics, including, for some people, helping alleviate chemotherapy's multiple side effects.

As reported in the **Journal of Ginseng Research**, a scientific publication chronicling research related to ginseng, an eight-week study conducted on human subjects, proved that Korean red ginseng (KRG) boosts immune functions. Compared to a placebo group, those participants given KRG experienced increased T-cells, B-cell antibodies, and other white blood cells. Additionally, observations indicate no adverse effects on those receiving KRG. A meta-analysis found that regularly consuming ginseng significantly decreases cancer risk, although the results are from laboratory tests, and more human studies are needed, including possible side effects and medication interactions. Yet, ginseng as a supplement may be beneficial.

Although turmeric is a spice well-recognized in health foods circles, I add it to my coffee, with coconut milk and honey; it is worth mentioning as a supplement. It is a rhizome, or underground stem; the purpose is to store nutrients for the plant to use during spans of deprivation such as winter and propagation of other plants. It is a spice typically used in Indian and Asian cooking. Its active chemical, curcumin, the active component used in most studies, is not very high in the spice alone. The most significant value is as an anti-inflammatory and antioxidant. Since many chronic diseases appear to be related to inflammation, turmeric may be an effective treatment for cancer and its reoccurrence.

The medical journal **Anticancer Research** focuses on experimental clinical subjects related to oncology. An article titled the **Potential Anticancer Properties and Mechanisms of Action of Curcumin**, discloses a correlation between the bioactive natural compound curcumin in turmeric and promising anti-cancer properties. Lab tests demonstrate potential anti-cancer attributes and cytotoxic effects on cancer stem cells. Its propensity to stop the spread of various cancer cell lines appears in breast, lung, oral, and colorectal studies.

An article in **Nutrients,** a journal on human nutrition, reports Curcumin's possible ability to target "...different cell signaling pathways including growth factors, cytokines, transcription factors, and genes modulating cellular proliferation and apoptosis." As a promising bioactive natural compound, it may be one of the most favorable anti-cancer supplements as a valuable accompaniment to standard cancer treatments. Its family member, ginger, traditional used to relieve nausea, which you may experience from chemotherapy, is also an anti-inflammatory that I drink as a tea, whereas I take turmeric in capsules. Warning: Ginger is generally considered safe, but some people have an allergy to it, and that may also cross over to turmeric since it is a relative.

Possible side effects experienced by some people include headaches, stomach upset, and diarrhea. Additional human studies are needed to understand its anti-cancer effects. Yet, I have elected to be the subject of my investigation by taking a supplement with a concentration of curcuminoids as a part of my daily routine. When selecting a turmeric supplement, be sure to look for the bioactive compound of curcumin and a black pepper root extract, as this is vital to the absorption of curcumin by the body.

A supplement that may be of value is vitamin A. Generally, a healthful diet will provide an ample supply of this antioxidant. Well-recognized as necessary to vision and skin, it also supports developing and maintaining T-cells that are part of a robust immune system.

One form of vitamin A that many of us are familiar with is retinol, a component of several skin care products, which occurs specifically in animal products such as fish. In comparison, plant foods are rich in vitamin A-promoting carotenoids, like beta carotene. A diet high in fruits and vegetables containing carotenoids helps protect against free radicals and oxidative stress, helping repair DNA damage and reducing the risk of chronic diseases, including some cancers.

A study appearing in **Cancer Science** noted that high levels of "...alpha-carotene and beta-cryptoxanthin (plant-related carotenoids) are associated with a lower risk of lung cancer death in US adults." Provitamin A carotenoids, αlpha-carotene, and beta-cryptoxanthin are converted to retinol in the body as a valuable form of vitamin A. Beta-cryptoxanthin has recently been cited in the **International Journal of Cancer** as potentially playing a role as a chem-preventative agent, opposing lung cancer.

BioMed Research International reviews documents of studies by experts in their field before publishing such research articles. It cites an investigation into the value of vitamin A derivatives in laboratory research. It notes a possible association between retinol and the reduction of the spread of some cancer lines, including breast and ovarian.

"Vitamin A strengthens your immune system by supporting white blood cells and the mucus membranes in your lungs, intestines, and urinary tract," according to the **Cleveland Clinic** online resource. Also, "...consuming higher amounts of beta-carotene or vitamin A from plant foods may protect against certain types of cancer." It is important to note that more information and additional human evaluations are necessary for a definitive answer to the value of vitamin A in the battle against cancer, while **The Journal of Immunology** indicates that deficiency in vitamin A in our diet has become a public health issue.

The best way to get any vitamin and mineral is in its natural form. Some of the best sources of vitamin A are cold-water fish like salmon and tuna, eggs with yoke, and bright-colored vegetables and fruits, such as carrots, sweet potatoes, avocados, mangoes, and others. But when diet alone doesn't provide them, supplements may be beneficial. Those most closely related to their natural form are the most absorbed by the body and, therefore, more helpful. The retinol form of vitamin A is in cod liver oil and beef liver, and both are available in gel capsules. Related to the cod liver, it can be taken orally directly as the oil (kinda nasty tasting). Beta-carotene, commonly found in retail supplements, is a plant based provitamin A that needs to be converted to retinol by the body to be effective. Studies suggest that vitamin A supplements of both varieties may assist the body in restoring valuable immune cells related to chronic disease and can play a role in fighting oxidative stress.

The last on this list is vitamin E. As with many vitamins and minerals, vitamin E is not just one compound but a class of potent fat-soluble antioxidants, with alpha-tocopherol being the most effective for humans. The best way to get this nutriment is through a healthful, balanced diet. Some top foods with it are nuts, seeds, cold water fish, avocados, red bell peppers, kiwi, and others.

Research indicates vitamin E's most significant benefit appears to be its ability to assist the body in dealing with oxidative stress, which occurs when there is an imbalance between free radicals and the body's ability to mount a defense against them. Oxidation left unchecked causes cellular damage, possible cell mutation, chronic and degenerative diseases, advances aging, and alters DNA. Medical science acknowledges that DNA corruption from oxidative stress significantly contributes to cancer development. Lifestyle habits like smoking, poor diet, and environmental exposures such as chemicals and pollution are all oxidative stressors influencing cancer development; hence, it is vital to control it.

Much of the investigative research on this vitamin centers around the ability to limit free radicals, thus preventing chronic diseases such as cancer. A 12-week randomized controlled trial, presented by the **National Institute of Health's Library of Medicine,** demonstrated that when compared to a placebo, supplemental vitamin E helps increase glutathione levels, the body's most potent antioxidant capable of protecting against cellular damage, removing toxins, and supporting immune functions and additional bodily operations. Because of vitamin E's antioxidant properties, it can improve kidney and liver functions, and with vitamin A, it can support eye health.

Vitamin E is most recognizable as an effective antioxidant, yet is multifunctional. Along with combating oxidative stress, it plays a role in the proper immune functions and is essential to cellular communications. It supports the immune system by promoting the increase of T-cells, or lymphocytes, a type of white blood cell critical to targeting pathogens, adaptive immunity, opposing cancer, and assisting other cells fight infection, enabling the body to boost the red blood cells it needs to carry oxygen through the blood for various functions like increasing energy.

When adding vitamin E and vitamin A in supplemental forms, be aware that both are fat-soluble. It is best to take them with fatty foods for the most significant absorption, but the body also stores them in fat tissue. It is essential not to consume excessive amounts of these, as they may accumulate in the body. In the case of vitamin E, it could exacerbate or possibly increase the risk of prostate cancer. The **Mayo Clinic** recommends 15 milligrams a day for adults. Be sure to consult your doctor before beginning a supplementation regimen with vitamin E because it may pose a safety risk for patients with a history of cardiovascular and liver problems, diabetes, and other conditions.

As a reminder, the value of most foods is not one specific factor. Instead, it is a compounding effect of many agents in them that promote good health and efficient bodily functions. Hence, it is vital to consume natural, wholesome foods. The benefits of vitamin E are valuable to helping you operate and feel your best, and this is why it may be necessary to use a supplement. Always ask your medical provider before augmenting your diet with outside additives.

Chapter 11

The Mind is a Terrible Thing ... To Waste

"A belief is not caused; it is created."
– Bruce Di Marsico

Many of you work with your hands in several different trades, or you spend your free time building and creating. Maybe it's a beautiful piece of furniture, rehabilitating a house, repairing things, creating incredible culinary dishes, developing a charming garden, or any other possibility—all requiring instruments and techniques to do so. Whether your employment is in this capacity or you do it with a personal sense of satisfaction, there are tools and skills necessary to complete the tasks. All are important to the process.

In integrative health, improving your diet and fitness are tools to advance your physical state. To integrate is to join; combining valuable tools for a better mind, body, and spiritual well-being is essential. The pursuit of peacefulness is one of those instruments. How one achieves will vary among people. Some find it in practicing their love of art. Maybe it's gardening or going for walks in natural settings. My friend

Joe, who has helped build and run a successful company and has two special needs children, retreats to his woodworking shop to relax. It is possible to find your zone of peacefulness.

Stress

Much research points to stress as a significant contributor to ill health. We are continuously under pressure, mental or physical; it is a normal part of life. The key is the response and adaptability to it. For instance, physical stress is how we build muscle. Challenging the body to do more physically causes a muscle to be damaged and break down. During the recovery, the body repairs itself and adds new muscle fibers, equating to added strength; this is positive stress. But when there is no recovery time for the body to rebuild from this stress, it becomes difficult to repair the damaged cells.

Just as a key to returning an injured area to balance and usefulness is rest, it is valid for the mind and emotional or psychological stress that can contribute to chronic ailments such as cancer. Studies have shown a relationship between chronic stress and DNA damage, the body's blueprint for healthy cell duplication of genetic material. This genetic information must be accurately copied and then assigned to new cells.

The **National Institute of Mental Health** studies the brain's biochemistry. The former director, Candace Pert, Ph.D., was one of the first to link the release of neuropeptides by the brain in response to emotions and stress and their effect on immune system function. She concludes that significant interaction exists between the molecules released by the brain because of emotions and stress and our physical health. Furthermore, they discovered that thoughts and feelings express themselves within the immune system. Her research awakens us to the consideration that there is a relationship between emotional responses, stress, and immune regulation.

A complex interplay between genes and the environment produces the effect of a gene having more than one expression or modifying how it exhibits as a consequence of emotions. As published in her article, "**Molecules of Emotion: The Science Behind Mind-Body Medicine**," Candace Pert, Ph.D., stated, "As our feelings change, this mixture of peptides travels through your body and brain. And they're changing the chemistry of every cell in your body." With this in mind, it is not unforeseen that emotions play a role in keeping the immune system healthy and balanced, as they influence the release of specific neuropeptides.

The immune system, a complex intertwining of several bodily functions and forces, is substantially disrupted by this emotional overload. Excessive cortisol, created by undesirable stress, causes an imbalance within these systems working together for good physical and mental health. Stress can arise from internal expectations of ourselves and those of others, and situations can result in frustration and tension within us and our relationships, leading to anger and even depression.

In the field of psychoneuroimmunology, a study of how what we think affects health, unfavorable expectations will eventually reveal themselves in various disorders. According to Mayo Clinic literature, negative thoughts, emotions, and behaviors can lead to stress. Without a way of releasing it, it can contribute to chronic conditions such as obesity, diabetes, and cancer. More than forty percent of us suffer from the adverse consequences of stress.

Persistent stress influences genetics, diet, environment, and lifestyle, and thereby our health. Stress exhibits itself in many ways. Physical symptoms may be insomnia, nausea, fatigue, discomfort in the gut, and a racing heart rate. Mental and emotional indications include crying for undetermined reasons, angry outbursts, depression, hopelessness, irritability, mood swings, and anxiety. Various behaviors from unfavorable stress may play a role in the destructive practices of drug and alcohol abuse, overeating, eating disorders, and social withdrawal.

The routine stress from my job, daily frustrations, financial challenges, irritation, and occasionally anger created by unwanted life situations and not living up to my expectations, I believe, were triggers for many internal reactions that eventually expressed as cancer. I knew I was in control of how to respond to stressful events and people, but I did not always implement that knowledge. Too often, I allowed my attitude about situations and others to move me toward a less empowered reaction. Some of this should have been short term, but sometimes I justified my righteous indignation, enabling situational stress to become chronic.

Oncologist Dr. Michael Hunter says, "How we manage stress has a crucial role in our physical and psychological well-being. Simple choices may yield powerful benefits." I often remind myself to focus on what I can do, and less on what I cannot do, helping me to be more positive. An enthusiastic mindset is among the best defenses against stress, leading to improved living.

Have you found positive strategies for managing stressful circumstances and relationships?

The key to effective stress management is identifying the things you can control and those you cannot. You can manage your actions toward your health, like diet, exercise, and rest. Choosing just one of these lifestyle areas, then adopting an improved habit, can be helpful. Combining several healthy habits will significantly lower stress levels.

Sometimes trying to do too much with too little time leaves us feeling overwhelmed or distressed. People over-schedule themselves and their children without including a period to wind down. A good way to reduce stress is to do less. Learn to say, "No can do," "Not going to do it," or "No." It's freeing and helps you to stay focused on what lifts your spirits, opening up the opportunity for a more positive view of life. Pick the most valuable things, then delegate lesser important things to others.

If you want a quick boost to your mental well-being, take a vacation from social media. Friendly public platforms sharing other's life experiences can be depressing when comparing their lives to ours. Many people I'm familiar with have expressed how much happier they were after giving up much of their social media. Connecting personally with friends and family is far better, as it creates stronger ties with those who can help us through stressful periods.

Can't resist the temptation to compare yourself to others? Maybe reflect on how fortunate you are when analyzing people's lives. I am lucky enough to see families traveling on airplanes, dealing with people who have life-threatening diseases or are born with physical impairments. As I observe their positive actions as they manage the needs of their children and others, I realize how blessed I am to have three healthy sons. Recognize all the incredible things for which you could be thankful. Developing an attitude of gratitude will assist in creating a more positive, happier psychology.

Most of us cannot go anywhere without a cell phone, "just in case." Some people sleep with it, because you never know who might ruin a restful night's sleep by needing to be the first to tell you the latest rumor, or how miserable life is. It is important to UNPLUG from the world during the evening. Most of what goes on can wait until later. I understand the value and peace of mind if your teenager is out or you have an impaired family member. Moving it away from your bedside so that each "ding" will not disturb you will improve your sleep. Explain to friends and family, when it is critical to speak with you, to call. The ringing will wake you up for important communications.

Life is a challenge; one thing you might find toughest to counter is one's reactions to events. There are times in the course of life when sh*t happens. It creates stress when we take things personally, as if it is there just to mess up our day. How you respond emotionally is the secret to the reaction by the body. Negative emotional expressions, like anger, increase the strain on the physical aspects of our bodies. Pausing and assessing the situation enables us to prioritize and set reasonable expectations for an acceptable outcome.

Do you want to feel better? Help yourself by choosing better options for managing stress. Identify in advance valuable choices for responding to stressful situations. There are various effective ways to take control of stress, while avoiding typical negative reactions of angry outbursts, excessive eating of comfort foods, smoking, alcohol and drugs, procrastination, irresponsibility, or, as many of us do, too much worrying.

A good place to start is the areas you have the most control over: diet and physical activity. These can be changed immediately, not only as a relief method but also as a preventative measure. Adopting a healthy lifestyle is a good starting point for stress reduction. I am sure the question, "What does diet have to do with stress?" is running through many people's minds. Woven together are the effects of the food we eat, our lifestyle, and how we deal with stress. Each affects our physical health and mental well-being. Some people are stress eaters. When they get overwhelmed, they find relief in food and drink. Seldom is a healthy bowl of blueberries or an avocado the choice. Instead, we choose comfort foods, a bowl of our favorite ice cream, chips, and such. These do not offer much nutritional value and lead to excessively useless calories, sometimes leading to becoming overweight and stressing the bodily systems.

Unhealthy eating habits associated with stress can lead to a lack of nutrients the body needs. Extended periods of stress change the physiological needs of the body. Metabolism rises with prolonged stress, increasing the use of many nutrients. If a person is nutritionally deficient, anxiety can worsen it, interfering with the body's ability to adapt to tension, and slowing recovery.

Creative, healthy ways that may serve you in relaxing can be walking, sitting in nature enjoying the surroundings, artistic endeavors, playing an instrument, singing your favorite mood-boosting or silly songs, finding ways to laugh, reading, taking a warm bath, deep diaphragmatic breathing, and other relaxation techniques. Make it a priority to take care of yourself so that you can be there to help family and others in need.

Yoga is effective for calming the mind while providing a workout. As one focuses on breathing and creating moments of mindfulness, it relieves stress. An article appearing in the **Journal of Clinical and Diagnostic Research** mentions that studies show reduced indications of internal inflammation are experienced by those who regularly practice yoga. As already discussed, chronic inflammation is linked to many protracted diseases, including cancer. A habitual yoga routine's advantages include better sleep, lower blood pressure, more mobility, improved balance, and other benefits.

Similar to yoga, Pilates is a relatively new form of exercise. Joseph Pilates developed it to help bedridden, wounded soldiers regain strength, stretch, and maintain muscle after World War I. These positive effects are through concentration, body and stability training, breath control, and proper joint alignment. All are to promote core strength and body awareness, enhancing physical and mental well-being. Where yoga has you center mentally to achieve peaceful well-being, Pilates has you focus on physical postures and motions to create a consciousness in the present moment.

Meditation

I am not an expert in the art of meditation. Yet, I believe there is an unwarranted sense that it is complicated. Even practicing simple forms like sitting in a quiet, relaxed, calming manner can have a positive effect. However, gaining the most benefits comes from making it a regular habit. Set aside time in your day, in the morning, at lunch, or before bed, and spend 15 or more minutes establishing a new practice of creating a center of tranquility. It will do wonders for your health.

Much evidence supports the concept of meditation as a helpful tool in calming and focusing the mind, making us less anxious, leading to more positive emotions, and generally being healthier. For example, there are cases of people, whose prognosis was expressed as incurable, going home, practicing meditation for extended periods each day, and incredibly becoming cancer-free. With nothing to lose, they embraced a victorious attitude. They transformed their disease and lives by changing their diets and daily habits and meditating to be at peace with their diagnosis, which became a catalyst for change that upgraded their outcome.

There are generally two simple types of meditation. One focuses on concentrating on something, ranging from an empowering scripture passage or prayer, an inspiring phrase, a tone or sound, like falling rain, a mantra or word(s), an image in your mind of possibly a positive experience, or simply breathing. The key is to keep it simple and pleasurable, creating a sense of relaxation. Focusing on one thing helps eliminate distractions from internal dialogue or noisy environmental inputs to the brain.

A technique that may be helpful is to start by taking a deep inhalation. Then let out a heavy sigh like you might express when being frustrated. Do this three or so times before relaxing into regular rhythmic breathing. Thinking and reciting a one-syllable word like one, love, calm, or any word that may help develop a feeling of relaxation is valuable. If your thoughts wander off to other areas of life, don't fret; return to thinking about your breath, keeping yourself centered in the present moment and away from stewing about the past or worrying about the future. It's that easy. Directing your thinking to what is happening right now can benefit your health.

While meditating, be careful to not let your mind take you down a rabbit hole of negative possibilities, leading to disempowering emotions that will not serve you. We've all experienced moments in our lives where we've spiraled downward from being unable to shake a negative memory, taking away empowering, desirable beliefs, and draining us of emotional and physical energy. Both these emotional and physical energies are needed to meet the challenges on the journey.

It's not so much about ignoring negative thoughts but more about not ruminating over past, unfavorable memories. It's important to recognize that we usually do the best we can with the experience and knowledge we have at that moment. Since you cannot change the past, it is better to learn from it to create a more enlightened and empowering future.

Many years of studies have demonstrated support of meditation as stress-reducing, thus improving immune system function. How it influences the body's bio-environment is complex and is being investigated continuously. However, many studies conclude that hypnotic-guided imagery, meditation, and mindfulness support a positive psychological response and a more robust immune system. Therefore, along with traditional therapies, incorporating these valuable tools as a part of an integrative plan can enhance a more favorable result.

Though exercising is an effective stress reliever and one I believe in, I still dedicate time for prayer and meditation. I often recite a prayer or scripture verses before I meditate, focusing on the scripture verses as I inhale and exhale, and giving me a sense of peace as I drift into a state of quietness. During some of these sessions, I received answers to questions I had asked while praying that day or a previous one. Each response was thought-provoking and put my mind at ease about the future, regardless of the outcome of my cancer journey.

Mindfulness

A type of meditation is mindfulness, which has become popular in the world of health and wellness. A quick explanation of mindfulness is to pay attention and appreciate life, our environment, and the activity around us, to be in the moment, an observer without judgment. Because when we judge, we recognize there is a choice of interpretation of an experience, and it is better not to be overly critical.

How we interpret past events and consider our future will affect our "now." Respect the past as inspiring lessons for today, and the future as stimulating possibilities. In the words of Thich Nhat Hahn, a Buddhist monk, "Do not lose yourself in the past. Do not lose yourself in the future. Do not get caught in anger, worries, or fears. Come back to the present moment, and touch life deeply." This is mindfulness.

Start as a spectator. Design more powerful moments by defining what is most important to you, and keep focused on those things you value, which is less about focusing on one specific vision or sound and more about appreciating the current moment, seeking to be aware of your surroundings and what's happening while not assessing thoughts as they pass through your mind. In the words of Kabat-Zinn, creator of the research-based program **Mindfulness-Based Stress Reduction**, it is "an awareness that arises through paying attention, on purpose, in the present moment, non-judgmentally."

Most of us have a mind full of all sorts of things, and they are generally non-inspirational. Mindfulness is taking time to quiet the conscious through awareness of the present moment, versus feeling overwhelmed with an overload of information. Most of the messaging and self-talk that fills our minds is negative. It is fed to us by an inexhaustive barrage of media platforms. Add concerns for our health, family members, finances, politics, work, and many other possibilities, and it is not surprising that anxiety and depression are on the rise, and when dealing with cancer, there is a bombardment of data. It becomes a mental strain, and we need a break.

Take the time to observe life and the energy of the moment, to pause and notice a thought or a feeling, mentally or physically. If you are curious about them, don't dwell on them. Say, "Hmm, isn't that interesting," and save the evaluation for another time. The goal of mindfulness is to arouse awareness of the subconscious processes taking place mentally, emotionally, and physically. A state of mindfulness moves the subject away from self-evaluation to just experiencing the present.

It is critical to recognize that your mind is a valuable instrument in an integrative approach to wellness. It can be an effective mechanism in helping you restore health and stay healthy, or it can be a hostile opponent—a way of making your mind your friend and not your foe can be accomplished through mindfulness meditation.

Teach yourself to be aware of thoughts, the feelings they generate, and sensations in your body. Don't be discouraged when the mind wanders. Acknowledge those ideas, then return your attention to your current place and time as often as it takes. Our society prides itself on multitasking, but research shows no such ability exists. It is just the shifting of focus from one task to another. You are never giving your full attention to a single effort. By my experiences, that sounds like "attention deficient" to me.

Train yourself to be a "monomaniac." I enjoy focusing on one task at a time, even when it is a more significant challenge than expected. My optimistic mind often gets me into projects that unexpectedly lead down a labyrinth of surprises, some difficult and others stimulating. Yet when I focus on one thing, it is far less frustrating than when I try to juggle many things simultaneously. My bride, Beth, is much better at that than I am, as are most moms.

I have found it to be incredibly challenging to live in the present. If you are in any way like me, past hurts, negative experiences, words, or failures pop back into your mind when positive inspiration is mainly needed. However, trying not to think about it has just the opposite effect. Neuroscientists have learned that we can't "not " think of something. Instead, we must replace it with new thoughts of what or who we want to become and focus on what is important right now. Creating affirming relationships, beneficial habits, and healthy lifestyle choices, and a good spirit, are solid foundational starting points.

I recall when I had achieved my dream of being hired by a major airline—a period in the industry when jet airplanes were less automated than they are today. A newly hired pilot was expected to understand the systems, how they worked, and what steps to take when things didn't go right, all by memory. Oh, yeah, and fly the plane. An instructor once told us that we received as much information in two weeks as a student would in an entire semester of college, and we were required to apply it correctly. It was challenging for a guy like me with attention deficit issues. Going from the start of training to being trusted with the flying public's safety took between six to eight weeks. Nevertheless, it is a fantastic feat that the airline industry training departments have mastered and continue improving upon while increasing safety.

During this time, an issue with a personal relationship occurred, adding to the mental demands of the tasks I faced as a newly hired pilot. At this time, the concept of compartmentalization became very useful. If you recall, compartmentalizing is putting life events into different boxes. Directing your attention to the present moment would be personal compartmentalizing, a type of mindfulness. Without it, I was destined to struggle and possibly fail. For this reason, it is encouraged by airlines and the FAA that pilots only fly when they are not distracted by life events, to be healthy in body, mind, and spirit.

Once you begin the practice of being mindful, the benefits will grow. Reducing the need to judge each event or person opens the door to new possibilities and flexibility for achieving dreams and desires, along with improved problem-solving. It helps to create a more relaxed mindset; thereby less stress. Fewer agitations enable us to handle life's trials and tribulations better. All these lead to improved, more powerful thinking, more restful sleep, lower stress and anxiety, reduced moments of depression, and less emotional and physical pain.

Try these practices if it is difficult to let go of the calendar, agendas, or worries, to center your focus on the present. First, schedule a short period of 5 to 15 minutes twice daily. My most valued moments are early in the morning, before the busyness of life begins, and just before going to bed, helping my mind to slow down. Whatever time you choose, making it a habit to set aside the time each day trains the mind to expect it, enabling it to come more quickly. Allow for the expansion of this period to grow to 20 or 30 minutes.

When choosing the best period for you, decide how and where to invest these moments:

- Sit quietly outside or in your favorite room
- Go for a leisurely walk
- Do yoga or other calming exercises like tai chi

Whatever you choose, decide to do the best you can to stay present. No scolding yourself is allowed when the focus unintentionally shifts away. Instead, gently bring it back, and commend yourself for being aware enough to recognize and return to the present moment.

During the day, hone your skills by directing your attention to one thing going on around you. If doing a task, recognize the sounds associated with it. For example, when you shower, listen to the water running, and observe how it falls through the air. Feel it running over your head and down your body and notice the different sensations as it caresses various parts. Is it warm? How does changing the temperature affect it? Hear it run down the drain and the shifting sounds. You may be thinking, "Dude, it's a shower." The idea is awareness of the accompanying perceptions individually, thereby practicing being focused on one thing each time.

Take the time right now and close your eyes. Find one sound to focus your attention on. How does it change as you listen? Does it grow louder or stay the same? Now try your sense of smell. What is unique? What is recognizable, pleasing, or not? If seated, what qualities does it possess, or when standing outside in bare feet, what does that feel like? Finally, name a positive feeling about yourself, and focus on the feeling it gives when used as an empowering tool to be your best. The key is to spotlight one thing at a time and appreciate all its associated attributes.

Mindfulness is keeping an intention as your center of attention. Therefore, appreciate each day more by filling it with all the amazing things that often go unnoticed. As we progress in the mindfulness habit, we learn to live in a state of mindfulness where life is marvelous. For a cancer patient or any life-threatening experience, this often begins as we recognize how valuable life is, leading to increased feelings of peacefulness, less negativity, better health, and relaxation. The key is to know, then choose the life you want, and be present in it.

We can plan for our future, yet we must live soulfully in the present. I say soulfully because to experience life to the max, you need to feel it emotionally, physically, and spiritually. The cancer journey has led me to believe that life is a spiritual adventure of becoming our best while assisting others to do the same. We influence others by how we live emotionally and the actions we take. I like the saying by Alice Morse Earle, an American author, and historian: "Yesterday is history. Tomorrow is a mystery. Today is a gift. That is why it is called the present."

There are many different ways to meditate or practice mindfulness. To get caught up in whether or not you are doing it right is defeating in nature. A simple form of creating a calm center is to direct your attention to your breathing. Be natural and relaxed. If you have ever watched a baby breathing while sleeping, you'll see their little belly raise slightly, then lower; this is natural, innate breathing—how we were created to breathe. Although the present is a twinkling of time, it will define your future.

Try this: Lying on your back or sitting comfortably in a chair, place a hand on your abdomen, and notice your breathing. Is it rising and lowering steadily? Natural breathing leads to a relaxed state. If it isn't rising naturally, or your chest is rising more noticeably than your abdomen, don't fret. You can train yourself to do it by focusing on causing the muscles in the midsection to expand and filling the lungs more fully with air, then relaxing those muscles, allowing the air to escape through your mouth and nose. With regular practice, it will become instinctive. At the same time, you are leading to a more relaxed presence.

According to Psychology Today's Gregg Henriques, Ph.D., mindfulness may arguably be "the single most significant development in mental health practices since the turn of the millennium." Considering our thoughts generate emotions and feelings, mindfulness is also valuable to managing mentally exhausting periods from dealing with cancer. Refraining from dwelling on the past or the future is incredibly challenging. I know. I'm a master at overthinking about both, often forgetting just how blessed I was and am now. I occasionally think and imagine how my life would have been different "if only...." "If only I would've or wouldn't have invested in that business," along with future "what if's." "What if my child chooses wrongly?" I was missing many delightful opportunities to experience "wow" moments. Realize how all the simply wonderful moments in life, from relationships to nature to sounds of birds, or even comfortable, pleasing imagery, can assist in promoting a healthy mind, body, and spirit.

One source stated that we spend 70 percent of our lives reliving past events and having anxiety about the future. Most of us expect that past events predict our future outcomes. Ruminating about our mistakes and worrying about things to come can lead to releasing the stress hormone cortisol, thus reducing immune function; when facing the uncertainty of a cancer diagnosis, stress and anxiety increase. But well-documented research has shown a reduction in stress hormone production in subjects who learned and practiced mindfulness and meditation.

The Society of Integrative Oncology suggests that increasing evidence supports the importance of meditation and other mind-body approaches, such as yoga or tai chi, as effective ways of dealing with chronic pain while reducing stress, anxiety, and insomnia. As a consequence, there will be improved mood and increased physical and emotional strength, balancing the mind-body-spirit connection and thus improving quality of life. The excellent part is that it is generally considered safe and health-enhancing, with positive side effects for any persistent condition, while easing the adverse byproducts of many cancer therapies.

Investigations into meditation by Perla Kaliman, who holds a Ph.D. in biochemistry and is a research scientist at **the University of California-Davis**, has revealed some of the effects of meditation on genes. As mentioned earlier, epigenetics is understanding that environment, diet, and lifestyle affect how our genes are expressed as a response to a stimulus. Preliminary small-scale studies suggest that directing attention to the present moments without judgment, which is what mindfulness and meditation are, may downregulate or decrease the expression of genes linked to inflammation, aging, and depression.

The health implications of meditation on physical well-being should steer science toward further investigations. Evidence that meditative-based training influences physical welfare warrants a thorough examination of existing information, as well as more studies on its power to impact gene expression. The consequences of mindful meditation related to chronic diseases, including cancer, healthy aging, and brain function, can act as guidelines for future analysis.

Now, take some time to sit in a rocking chair, on a park bench, at the beach, or someplace where you can be an observer. Let the moment fill your senses. Listen, smell the aromas, see the colors and be a spectator of actions, an uncritical people watcher, feel a breeze moving across your skin, and enjoy the taste and texture of ice cream; there are some good non-dairy ones also. The idea is learning to appreciate the little things we have taken for granted.

Spiritual

I do not judge people on their connection with universal intelligence, a divine creator, or if they even have any belief in a greater power. Individual events can lead us toward or away from a chosen attitude. Through personal investigations and life experiences, I believe there is more beyond this earthly existence. If I am wrong, I will never know the difference. If I am right, I will always experience the difference. My belief is partially built on, as modern physics has explained, the fact that energy cannot be created or destroyed.

Besides this understanding, no one in science has been able to explain simply enough for me to "get it," without some guiding force, how a complex symbiotic culture like the human body could develop by random chance. Albert Einstein is credited with the comment, "If you cannot explain it to a six-year-old, then you don't understand it yourself." I do not feel badly about not understanding a genius's reasons why random selection is how everything came into existence, since like me, you're at least as bright as a six-year-old.

Many of us have questions running through our minds, such as, why did this happen to me? What did I do to deserve this? Why is God punishing me? We are in a low emotional state when we ask these questions. I was troubled by such inquiries as these to the divine. Through praying, meditation, and conversations with clergy, I understand a medical condition may result from a chosen lifestyle, diet, environment, and some genetics, but not divine retribution.

The development of a chronic condition like cancer surprises people and their families. It brings us to the realization that life is unpredictable, especially when we believe we have done all the right things. Please do not allow a disease to become your identity. It is psychologically beneficial to consider these as just events in life. If you talk about the condition of cancer, avoid owning it. It's not "your" cancer. It is just cancer. It just so happens that a combination of conditions enabled it to become established in your body.

Events such as persistent afflictions lead us to re-evaluate what matters. It opened my eyes when I reflected on the possibility of not being around for my family and their needs. For most of my life, it was meaningful for me to have the respect of others and for people to believe in me as I do in myself. I am not sure where that mindset developed, but I think it came about when I heard many times when I was young, something like, "You can't do that" (the source was not my parents), suggesting I was not capable. All of this has changed through living life as I no longer care what others think. What matters is what I believe to be possible for myself. Yet, I still contemplated whether Beth could provide for our sons in the manner I conceived. Who would guide them to be the best man possible without an example to follow? Assuming my actions were worthy of adoption, these types of questions were more troublesome for me than the disease itself.

My new focus was on what I could do and how to show my family, and anyone observing, not to give up but to live with a purposeful, positive attitude as I ran the race for my life, physically and mentally. I learned that all I can do today is enough. So tomorrow, I will do whatever I can, each day. For me, to win was to not let cancer take my spirit. That became the example I wanted my boys to understand, as well as how to live their lives with a sense of joy and amazement.

There are days when just getting through it is all you can manage, which is okay. "Tomorrow, tomorrow, there is always tomorrow," as the song goes. Of course, long-term survival is the objective, but thriving at the moment is what you want to achieve daily, especially during the challenging times. By staying directed towards whatever you can do every day, with diet, physical activity, and mental and emotional inputs, improving your lifestyle provides a sense of control and is morale-boosting.

A good day can be encouraging enough to keep a condition from dominating you emotionally as you strive for better health. Sometimes, it is necessary to find a minor thing to improve your mood. I recall a series of days when I felt incredibly uncomfortable in the area of my stomach. After eating breakfast one morning, I sat in a rocking chair outside the Transplant House in Rochester, MN, when suddenly I got the urge to heave. I arrived in the washroom just in time to enjoy my breakfast a second time as it passed through my mouth and into the toilet. But I felt much better. The discomfort in my gut was gone, enabling me to get outside and savor a glorious spring day. As crazy as it sounds, regurgitation upgraded my experience that day and became my victory. Sometimes, highlighting the good in the little things can distinguish between a positive and gloomy outlook. Own your day by finding success; regardless of how small or silly, you can claim it. It may be the modest wins that keep us believing in more significant possibilities.

Seeking a sacred experience with the divine is a possible way to define spirituality. In addition, the appreciation of life's purpose, beyond purely physical, can offer health benefits, including lower stress. Research, published in the **International Journal for the Psychology of Religion**, reports those who follow a religious doctrine have a more relaxed demeanor, leading to improved mental health, lower substance abuse, and generally longer, happier lives.

A common phrase in society is, "I am spiritual but not religious." I have uttered these words myself. A spiritual connection beyond our mere existence provides a sense of purpose and guidance, yet being involved in a similar community of people is life-enhancing, according to a **California Public Health Foundation** study. An evaluation of individuals, covering almost three decades, found a strong relationship between reduced mortality and participation in religious services. An additional analysis published in the **American Journal of Public Health,** on a study following 1931 seniors, supports an association between longevity and religious observances. How or why does this occur?

Possible explanations may be related to theological principles that promote better health by abstaining from excessive substance use and having more positive lifestyle habits and stress-reducing practices. People with a belief in a higher power may be able to find meaning in traumatic life events. Yet, many not affiliated with an organized faith follow such health-enhancing routines, and their life span is shorter than those involved in a religious community. Being actively engaged in a spiritual community may extend one's life from seven to 14 years. These groups of people tend to have lower blood pressure and cardiovascular disease, a more positive demeanor, reduced rates of suicide, improved immune functions, and a lower rate of cancers.

Caution: Choosing to follow a disheartening religious dogma that stimulates thoughts of guilt, shame, or fears of retribution from God, may cause a mental and physical stress response, leading to poor health. The key is a positive spiritual experience within a religious community providing a personally empowering state of mind, allowing you to find comfort and divine inspiration in overcoming the disease. The support, hospital visits, and prayers from my and Beth's church members (we belong to different affiliations) were encouraging. I was appreciative of their interest and concern for my well-being. With all those positive vibes flying around, I felt some had to land on me.

But truthfully, one of my spiritual beliefs is that positive energy begets positive influences. The opposite is also accurate. Regular exposure to negative inputs or dark energy (not the space kind) can adversely impact life, which is readily recognizable in society and is often used by the media to sway public opinion because it is more sensational than finding positive events, and you usually find more of what you focus your attention on. Be a good finder and see abundance in the world. Be a faultfinder and there will be plenty of opportunities to place blame for the world's problems. I prefer to live with an attitude and a God of abundance, and the freedom that comes with a positive outlook, and believing good can be found in the craziness.

A spiritual skill to develop that can promote positive health benefits is the concept of forgiveness. I think it is safe to say that most religious doctrines teach that a key to peace in life follows an attitude of forgiveness. But it goes beyond a religious dogma and is even recognized by modern psychology as essential to flourishing in the areas of happiness, health, relationships, and all aspects of well-being.

Forgiving is not forgetting, but more of shifting focus forward to the present. Anger and resentment are two powerful negative emotions that keep us living a painful past and can prevent us from building an empowering future. Choosing a positive emotion like forgiveness, enables you to live a more fulfilling life with an increased sense of freedom and self-worth. Paul Boese said it well, "Forgiveness does not change the past, but it does enlarge the future." The value of forgiveness is recognized as being a life enhancing practice that pays the greatest benefit to the forgiver. Leave the past where it belongs—behind you—and learn from it and then look forward as you travel on the road ahead.

In all your forgiving, be sure to forgive yourself as well, for past actions, or lack thereof, and mistakes made. Acknowledge and accept responsibility for misunderstandings, but don't possess them. Personally, I can pass harsh judgement on myself, but self-condemnation is of no value to health, and it offers no long-term benefit. Personal forgiveness is a small, yet empowering step towards emotional healing and primes us for determining ways to respond positively in the future. Have patience with yourself and lapses in the efforts to release blame. It takes practice. It is easier to start with small misdeeds to let go of, before focusing on bigger ones that may take longer. Always remember that learning from an experience is valuable to preventing a reoccurrence, while positively moving forward.

There are many types of relaxation techniques, from paying attention to your breathing, to focused meditation techniques, to regular prayer and habits of gratefulness and forgiveness, each with the intent of helping reduce stress. Though these are traditionally thought of as mind enhancing, evidence supports the concept that what is good for the mind reflects favorable in the body.

Chapter 12

Attitudes are Contagious, Catch a Good One

"Attitude is a little thing that makes a big difference."
– Winston Churchill

If you're like me, when you received the diagnosis of cancer, possibly one of the first mental responses was something like, "Why me?" Shifting my focus away from this helpless thinking to a more forward-looking idea of, "What am I going to do about it?" changed my stress level.

Choosing a victor's mentality over the victim's approach is effective in any facet of life, especially with cancer. A victim receives the diagnosis and assumes that only modern medicine can fix it—"I'm just along for the ride" psychology. On the other hand, you can choose a victory or winning mindset of, "I may have cancer, but I'm not going to let cancer have me," as you walk this incredibly challenging path. Rediscovering a willingness to do whatever it takes to beat it, may be the decisive turning point in your life and how you handle cancer.

The concept that you can influence how this disease affects you can transform the experience. Deciding you have the best chance at advancing or enduring in this time of physical corruption by taking actions that give you the best odds of winning or beating this chronic condition, may alter the consequences of the treatments; whereas perceiving that there is nothing you can do about it—helplessness or victimhood—you will be more likely to tolerate what you get. You deserve more than just surviving. Decide that thriving is where you want to go.

Researchers have found a direct relationship between your mental mindset and the effects of a disease. How a patient responds to the trauma of an illness can leverage the body's release of hormones and will impact the heart, digestion, and respiratory system while influencing an immune reaction. Our attitude and core beliefs are critical to mental and physical health, including how the body deals with cancer.

Mindset plays a significant role in the creation of neuropeptides and their release by the neurons or nerve cells. These peptides drive and mediate multiple regulatory functions involving organ systems, including the immune complex, balancing intercellular communications between our neurology and the endocrine operations. As published in her article, **"Molecules of Emotion: The Science Behind Mind-Body Medicine,"** Candace Pert, Ph.D., stated, "As your feelings change, this mixture of peptides travels through your body and brain. And they're changing the chemistry of every cell in your body." With this in mind, it is not unforeseen that emotions play a role in keeping the immune system healthy and balanced, as they influence the release of specific neuropeptides. These chemical messengers create a feedback loop amid organs and the glands that manufacture and manage their release. This system can be "messed up" by environmental chemicals, lifestyle, and stress.

After an 80-year study, it is determined and recorded in the book, *The Longevity Project,* that for people with a habit of expecting the worse when faced with challenging situations, their pessimistic assumptions appear to become exacerbated. These tendencies make them less likely to take actions that can influence a positive outcome. Lack of effort may increase frustration and depression. Yet, **Leslie Martin, Ph.D.,** of **La Sierra University**, states, "Many people who lived through hard times went on to live long lives," applying what they learned to deal with their predicament.

Those who considered their diagnosis a source of motivation, establishing meaning in these circumstances, seem to benefit from this perspective, leading them to create regular practices, promoting a healthy body and mind. Yet, how one emotionally handles hardships is arguably as valuable as daily habits like exercise, a quality diet, and stress reduction. Conscientiously attacking your plight with an integrative plan can strongly predict your persistence in your efforts to be victorious.

Your belief in what is possible is essential. It will either spur your mind to adopt a catastrophic view, causing rumination and worry, or to see an event as a need for a lifestyle change. Depending on which perspective you accept, will shape your actions. For example, taking an active role by adopting new eating habits, exercise routines, and mindfulness methods shifts the idea of cancer from a fate-filled outcome to a disease with a chance of victory.

Studies indicate that the best protection against diseases, including cancer, is an empowered mindset that develops when we believe we influence our outcomes. Many people have overcome their addictions, ill health, lack of money, and others, by looking at these as opportunities to change. Change is growth, which is valued psychologically, spiritually, and physically. Discovering and putting your most authentic values to work will enhance your confidence, relationships, and emotional and physical feelings. Together they can positively change your health.

What you believe to be true can be more important than reality. Assumptions lead us to make decisions in one direction or another—my experience from when I broke my neck formed within me an understanding that mindset matters. The desire to not accept my circumstances as they appeared, partial paralysis, motivated me to not give in to ruinous thinking. Feeding my mind with positive ideas helped me believe in myself and stay focused on my dream of flying the big jet airliners, which I realized at age 25.

Believing the body is an incredible biome that continuously adapts to its environment, promotes more positive emotions for managing fears, events, and a better quality of life. **The Journal of Clinical Oncology** says, "Focusing on the psychological and social elements of the cancer experience can alter both functional and disease-specific outcomes." Your mindset matters. Nourishing the desire to live life to the fullest will push you forward to be a victor over a disease.

Are you a cancer victim, or is it a catalyst for change? Whatever meaning you give will push you in the direction of actions or inaction. In the branch of medicine of psychoneuroimmunology, studies of the effects of the mind on health and resistance to disease, it has been demonstrated that there is a correlation between our emotional reactions to life's difficulties and the immune system's response to a disorder. A given neurological response will release hormones into the body, activating the nervous system. An affirming counter to a situation or disease, a person helps deliver happy hormones or neurotransmitters of dopamine and serotonin, producing oxytocin. In return, you will experience positive emotions, relaxation, and other psychologically stabilizing feelings.

On the other hand, when we experience a negative or stressful situation, the nervous system releases noradrenaline and cortisol to prepare us to defend ourselves or flee, the classic fight-or-flight response, which many of us are familiar with. Though this systematic response by the body enables us to survive encounters with the natural elements of our world, the body will have the same reaction regardless, even if the experience is only emotional. It can't tell the difference between a physical threat and a mental or psychological one. The problem is that releasing these chemical substances affects the immune system, creating inflammation. When noradrenaline and cortisol enter the blood, they block nature killer cells rather than letting them attack foreign bodies and rogue cells within us. Just one of the ways an optimistic approach to life can benefit us.

There are numerous accounts of people who overcame insurmountable odds or defied what the masses thought was possible to overcome cancer disease. So be conscious of the "expert's" statistics. You are not a number but a unique individual. Statistical statements can be damning. Don't own them.

Instead, challenge yourself to live your life filled with a determination to do all you can through actions, diet, lifestyle, treatments, and mindset. I dare say, for every cancer type, someone has beaten the odds. No one knows your outcome, and it is wrong for anyone to lump you into a group of numbers. The statement, "You have X amount of time to live," has caused some to prepare for death. In contrast, others have formulated a plan to live life to the fullest.

One study looked at incurable metastatic cancer patients. In the publication **Clinical Cancer Research**, it was reported, patients who adopted a personal center of control towards the disease and embraced a self-healing concept, lived longer than the medical experts or the numbers projected. If a doctor appointment ends with, "There is nothing that can be done." I encourage you to find another opinion. There is always something, like improvement in mental, spiritual, and physical practices.

Whether positive or negative, your view of life affects how successful you will be in the endeavors you pursue. Seeing life as a series of events trying to stop us from having what we want will lead to the belief that we are victims of our heritage, environment, health, and many other possibilities. It's not uncommon to find people from the same environment, family, company, and so on, yet one lives an abundant life while another is struggling.

You may be familiar with siblings who grew up in a family wherein a parent had a substance abuse problem. One of them vowed never to touch the stuff and to get away from the atmosphere in which they grew up. But, unfortunately, the other falls into the same lifestyle and adopts the negative habits they experienced during their upbringing, then blames it on genes or the environment they grew up in. One sibling used the experience as fuel for motivation to seek change for the better, while the other considered the past as a weight, drag, or brakes holding them back.

The question is, which perspective would you choose? A prudent choice is to empower yourself by taking action toward positive change. A positive choice creates a greater sense of "I can handle it" or adaptability. Without believing in yourself and the ability to adjust and move forward, one is more likely to look for others to solve their challenges. By seeking to blame or rely on someone else or an organization as to why we are where we are, or are not where we want to be, we relinquish control of our happiness to others.

Do I believe having a positive mental attitude will cure you? Nope. I want to make it clear; it could be fatal if one thinks beating cancer is simply mind over matter. But with a positive approach, you'll accomplish more and avoid the trap of victimhood. I want to emphasize that our emotional states affect the body's chemistry. The field of psychoneuroimmunology is now exploring the link between the frame of mind and health.

It is crucial to emphasize that your mental focus and your positive or negative mindset will influence your actions. Therefore, your psychology is a component of your treatment. As personal development leader Tony Robbins has said, "Where focus goes, energy flows." Your decision to choose positive behaviors will affect the quality of your experience. It may determine the outcome.

Taking constructive action and doing your part affirms that you have some control over this trek. Gathering information and learning as much as possible reframes how you respond to the diagnosis. Applying your newfound knowledge can help diminish stress and anxiety and may curtail depression. Creating a plan that you can implement is vital to controlling emotionally challenging life events, while establishing healthy habits to deal with the pressure of this epic experience can be immune boosting.

Observations of natural killer (NK) cells in breast cancer patients are shown to be more active in women with a more positive, action-oriented psychological state than those who felt helpless. Dr. Ron Herberman, MD, at the **University of Pittsburgh Cancer Institute**, noted an increased activity of NK cells, improving prospects of life continuance. Research in Japan confirms these results.

Susan Lutgendorf of the **University of Iowa** confirmed similar results with ovarian cancer in women. The patients with strong emotional support and who felt loved were able to keep a more positive spirit. This group had higher numbers of NK cells than those distressed and feeling helpless. Evidence supports the perception that white blood cells of the immune system perform most effectively when the host believes in the ability to govern their attitude.

It's not just about having a positive attitude versus having a negative one. More importantly, it is believing in the abilities to construct a more favorable response to the disease; that is what makes the difference. Much research indicates that our immune system is especially sensitive to emotions of helplessness. Consistent feelings of powerlessness affects the body's reaction to a disease, whereas a strong desire to win, or not give up, becomes a point of decisive change in the course of the disease.

Reframe

I have chosen to believe that life's events are constantly testing us; not to kick dirt in our faces but to kick us in the butt to move forward and to grow. It is only through these mental evolutions that we become adaptable. One of the greatest attributes one can possess to empower them to be their best is adaptability. Investigate anyone who has worked to achieve a dream, desire, or goal; you will find this quality of adjusting to situations an endearing trait. The essence of the heart, mind, and spirit's passion for living lies in the belief that we can learn from experiences, then build upon them a foundation for a means of a rewarding life.

Regardless of finances, social standing in the world, IQ, political persuasions, or whatever sense of a higher power you believe in, there are problems and difficulties. The graveyard is the only place on this planet where there are none of the stressful dilemmas of life we all deal with. Those people have no problems and no life.

Each of us has a choice to make in our ideology. One is "life is unfair," or "why me?" I'll be the first to admit that life is not fair. It's not. A young mother has her life taken by cancer, leaving a family behind without the loving, caring spirit of giving that a mother offers. It's unjust that a blossoming child's life is snuffed out by disease, violence, or abuse. It is cruel that these things happen. Actions are necessary to end such incidences in every case. Begin with what we can control: our beliefs and behaviors. Adopt a new attitude of turning stumbling blocks into building blocks.

Another possibility is to perceive that life doesn't play favorites. It is what it is, as the famous saying goes. What if we condition ourselves to believe that the more challenges we face constructively, the more we grow toward being our best? Transform your thinking to see living as just a series of experiences, choosing to accept them as growth enhancing or as restraints on you being the best you can be. Allowing for the possibility that we are capable of more than our current expectations, empowers us to say to ourselves, "Why not me?" There is no reason I can't ethically achieve my aspirations "if" I am willing to give enough to be who I say I want to become.

An attitude of, "If I desire it badly enough, then I will do whatever it takes to achieve it or experience it," is a benefit. I want to emphasize "whatever it takes" versus "anything it takes." The word "anything" lends itself to meaning it's acceptable to break the law or at least act in an immoral, unethical manner, whereas "whatever" recognizes boundaries. Your health, integrity, and character are more important than "getting" a prized possession or aspirations of a particular social economic level of living. Will you get precisely what you want? To paraphrase the famous modern-day philosopher Mick Jagger, "You may not get what you want, but if you try, sometimes you get what you need." I've learned that lofty goals move us forward in the right direction. Maybe we don't realize what we envisioned specifically in our dreams, yet we still live a fulfilling life that started in our imagination, even in small doses.

Ask Better Questions

Here are some of the beneficial concepts I found helpful as alternatives to the discouraging feelings I was experiencing. First, it is imperative to recognize this cancer stuff has invaded your body. I know what you are thinking: "Duh, that's helpful." One of the things you need to avoid is the "why me" syndrome—asking God or the universe, "Why did this happen to me?" It does nothing to fix the challenge you face. Be confident, knowing it is not a punishment for a fall from grace.

Okay, it is what it is. Now, a better question is, "What can I do to improve my health." Or "How can I use this and be better at being me?" Answering such questions provides you with a sense of power. To conceive a winning game plan, one must feel the strength of personal authority over one's world. Otherwise, it is paving the way to victimhood.

It is also important not to become angry over the fact that cancer is now part of a newfound reality. Neither anger nor victimhood is helpful, and neither is wishfully hoping, which many confuse as having a positive attitude.

Instead, a solid, constructive response is deciding to become informed and learn how to help yourself and improve your odds of winning. Having a positive approach is not denying what you are experiencing. Instead, it's choosing to be a problem solver. Understanding, to the best of one's abilities, the situation and how to overcome it through personal effort while integrating it with medical technology, is fundamental to overcoming a pessimistic state of mind, enabling a conquering of your plight. In turn, it serves as a way to defeat helplessness, which is what makes you a victim instead of a victor in any capacity.

In the Hebrew testament of the Bible, the book of Proverbs tells us that if we focus on the lions in the jungle, we won't step outside for fear of being a victim or being killed. Envisioning the worst stops us from taking action and surrendering to circumstances and outside forces to determine our fate, sapping any liveliness within us and moving away from the person we know in our hearts we are capable of becoming.

What's Great About a Positive Attitude

One of the attributes that come with developing a positive attitude is being mentally tough. Recalling when I had the task of providing a eulogy when my mother died, I contemplated what I would say. So many thoughts came to mind as I compared the personalities of my mother and father and how they shaped our family.

I always wanted to be like Dad—a big man, six feet two inches tall, with a chest like a barrel. I once watched him carry a full-size refrigerator up a flight of stairs on his back—a man who, by his presence, drew respect from others. But, of course, with things turning out the way they sometimes do, the only thing I physically inherited from my father was his muscular composition.

On the other hand, my mother was a petite woman who, maybe at her peak, was five feet two inches. Both my parents had a fantastic work ethic and a determination to do whatever was needed to take care of their family, which was very demanding, with seven children plus the two of them.

As I remember them, their likeness, and differences, one of the attributes my mother had was a positive, caring attitude. At one point, we moved in with our aunt and grandmother when my father made a career change and money was limited. Mom was taking care of Grandma, who was all but bedridden, babysitting the first grandchild while her parents worked, and Mom was employed part time to help pay the bills while still seeing to the needs of her children. As I looked back, it occurred to me that my mom was a mentally tough woman.

I believe developing a positive attitude is rooted in mental toughness. When life steamrolls you with a cancer diagnosis or any life confrontations, will you choose to be a victim and accept fate, or will you say, "Hell no!" and decide by your actions and attitude not to let it defeat you mentally while battling it physically?

Life is chocked full of adversities. Cancer patients generally fall into physical, mental, emotional, social, and spiritual categories. Each area presents challenges to keep the disease from getting the best of you. Facing each challenge as they come, sometimes more than one at a time, creates feelings of empowerment. Recognizing that you are in control of how you respond to adversity is a crucial step on the journey of a victor. Winning comes by knowing there will be difficulties, then dealing with them.

Though diagnosis is usually factual, based on science and the medical community's experiences, prognosis, or the predicted results you can achieve personally, is speculation. It is an attempt to forecast or, worse, conclude your future. Each of us is different genetically, physically, mentally, and spiritually. Therefore, no person truly knows the prospects and what you, or the human body and mind, can do.

I am of the personality type that may be defiant, but I use it positively. When someone says, "you can't," I ask, "why can't I?" Then I explore how to realize my desires. Some dismiss me, or they label me with their opinion, like "Napoleon complex" (I'm not tall). I've never knowingly used that as a reason or motivation to do or become anyone I wanted. But even if I did, so be it, because it has served me in achieving many of my heart's desires, including winning over cancer.

Ancient beliefs are in the lore of various native peoples in different lands. One that is crazily wild to me has its roots in the aboriginal people of Australia. There was an act in some tribes referred to as "the pointing of the bone." It consisted of a ritual ceremony to bring an affliction to a member by pointing a magical bone at the victim while uttering a curse by a shaman. The marked person would fall ill and eventually die. There is evidence of its effectiveness, as well as the reversal of the condition.

Two preconditions must have existed for it to be effective. First, the victim must know that they are cursed. Next, they must believe in the culture with absolute acceptance of the lore and power of the bone. All was brought about by believing in the shaman's authority and ability to affect a person's health by pointing this bone and uttering words. Voodoo spells cast by a "witch doctor" operate under the same preconceived principles of belief.

That's ludicrous, you might be thinking. Is it? Have you ever listened to someone describe their experiences of a particular illness, then compare your symptoms and begin feeling poorly yourself because they seem similar? I have seen it happen. It's not inconceivable for medical students to acquire the symptoms of the disease they are studying. The words spoken to us by a person we believe to be an authority influence us positively and negatively, regardless of the accuracy of their statements.

According to Doctor Ian Gawker, a modern-day shaman could be our doctor, whose prognosis may be the pointing of the bone. He argues that a poor prognosis can lead to battling two illnesses, cancer and the patient's belief that their fate is predetermined. He includes that trying to predict the outcome is like the "odds on a sporting event. The favorite often wins, but there are times they don't."

Living in Kentucky, there are many opportunities to go to horse racing events. To make it more exciting and fun, when I go, I try picking and betting on the horses by looking at the history of each one. But history alone doesn't predict the future with certainty. I've learned that the favorite is only sometimes the winner. Track conditions, the other horses, the jockey, and many other influences can affect the results. The formula for determining which one will come in first uses statistical analysis, yet each race is unique.

As each horse and race is unique, so are you. You and cancer are not a statistical event. You are unique. We are, individually, genetically, chemically, and mentally different. That is why not every treatment works for every person. For example, Revlimid, a medication for multiple myeloma, was ineffective for me, while other patients benefited from its use. An approach of one-size-fits-all cannot create an extraordinary outcome. My experience is that I can influence the odds of the result by adapting and adopting a new diet, lifestyle, and a determination to win over cancer.

One of the reasons why having a positive mental toughness is vital is that it will empower you emotionally. How you feel mentally becomes a driving force that will either charge you with a desire not to give up the fight or to surrender to the strenuous assault taking place physically and psychologically. Take steps to care for your needs physically, mentally, and emotionally, regardless of how you feel bodily. Meeting personal needs in these areas will strengthen your resolve in this journey. Go further than you think you can, even if it's just one more step.

Research has shown a persistent attitude of helplessness affects the body's response to illnesses, including cancer. In comparison, those that take action have the best rate of survival. If I have led you to believe I think it's all mental, I want to emphasize a positive attitude is not a cure. Think of positive mental toughness as a way to navigate a road with its twist and turns, potholes, hills, and dips along a path; not as a superhighway to your destination. An affirming constructive approach to life doesn't allow you to succeed at everything but enables you to do everything better than having a negative attitude.

My experience has been that it is far better to believe in the positive possibilities than to become miserable by accepting someone else's input unchallenged. If you are not careful, continuous negative vibes from the outside world, including the medical community, will make you believe you are just another casualty of cancer. We are about being victors and not living as a victim. You are the person who you are working on becoming: healthy, joyous, peaceful—a life-affirming individual. Being the best you can be at the moment, leads to peace of mind.

Developing Positive Mindset

So how do we shift a negative attitude to focus more on positive possibilities? To start, reread the spirituality, meditation, and mindfulness section, and emphasize living in the present—practice mindfulness thinking. Avoid looking back at past missteps or having too much anxious future thinking. Instead, remember to learn from the past, yours and others, plan, not worry about the future, and be in the present and have the quality of life accompanying the appreciation of sharing.

The key to creating the best possible outcome lies in embracing the challenge of the road before you. As the saying goes that the elite warriors of the U.S. Navy Seals adopted, "Embrace the suck!" Committing to doing all you can opens up the positive potential of the mind, spirit, and body. A belief in the best possible outcome will only come with positive, hopeful, emotional expectations of winning over the experience of cancer.

Start escaping unfavorable, fearful programming by letting go of social media. What started as an excellent way to keep in touch with friends and family has become politicized, a platform to attack people or attempts by some to outdo others. The snarky comments accompanying some of these posts, or the tendency to compare our lives with others that may grow from viewing such items, are defeating in nature. These are not life-enhancing but emotionally diminishing, undermining a valuable aspect of winning in any area of your life; health is one of them. If you are afraid to drop social media platforms altogether, start by limiting your exposure time to one day a week. I know people who began this way and now view it on limited occasions and are much happier.

One valuable thing to do is avoid the statistics. You are not a number; giving too much attention to them can lead to anxiety and despair. Some may say you need to be more realistic. I say winners aren't. They don't stop with what is but rather stay engaged in the process by doing all they can do without the concerns of what they can't do. They keep going one step at a time to discover what is possible. There is always something you can do, even if it is only being able to pray and find peace. Peace is only genuinely available through positive prayer, meditation, and mindfulness. These reduce stress. Less stress, less cortisol. Less cortisol, less inflammation—inflammation being a promoter of cancer and its spread.

Gratefulness

A life-affirming practice that has received considerable recognition in recent years is the practice of gratefulness. Taking the time to account for the many things we have to be thankful for is a practical step in becoming more positive. It helps us re-examine our world and the abundance that fills our lives. I am often reminded of this when I visit the Mayo Clinic and reflect on the many people, I see they're dealing with personal ailments or those of another cherished person. It's my wake-up call to how blessed I am with my health, an incredibly supportive wife, and that I have three healthy sons and helpful brothers, sisters, and friends.

It is beneficial to acknowledge those things we are grateful for—the natural beauty of a sunset, trees, flowers, or a relationship, clean water to drink, and the warmth of a coat on a windy winter day. I've heard many variations of how people practice gratitude, from keeping a thanksgiving journal, meditating on what they are grateful for, and including it in their dinner table prays. There is a myriad of possibilities. I am not sure whether writing them down is of greater importance than an act of appreciation. I'm one to do what easily flows and is relaxing. I'll take time to sit quietly and review my day to find things that are useful or valuable. Sometimes, I lie in bed at night, realizing it escaped me, so I give thanks at that time.

The value of recording things is the ability to look back and reflect on what you have written down. Sometimes, we need to get through some tough times, and being able to refresh a memory will pull oneself out of the doldrums. What's important is learning to honor life, the people in it, the endowment of personal talents, the freedoms we enjoy, and the sacrifices others have made for our benefit. Be sure to include the challenges that shape and change us. By making this a habit, you soon develop an appreciation for each day. You'll discover more things to be happy about, setting a positive foundation to build powerful habits for a more rewarding life.

It is optional to wait until the end of the day. One of my favorite times is early in the morning. I like to sit on our deck with a cup of coffee, listening to the birds welcoming the dawn of a new day. I'll give thanks for that moment, my health, how blessed I am to live surrounded by nature, the sleep I got, and whatever comes to mind. When in chemotherapy, I was satisfied that I didn't "toss my cookies." I follow that with affirmations of gratefulness. These may go something like, "I am so happy and grateful that I am or have...," and fill it in with many possibilities, such as good health or a future personal development goal. For example, while I was writing this book, it was, "I am so happy and grateful that I can write a book and help people become their very best and a force for good and empowerment throughout the world. Thank you." Finding things to appreciate at the start of the day primes me for a better mood, encourages me to work on my goals and desires, seeks positivity, and sets the stage for a more gratifying day.

Beginning and concluding the day with gratefulness in your heart leads to living more self-affirmingly, inspiring the building of constructive habits, and a greater appreciation for the simplicities of life; in turn, bringing about increased happiness. This is especially true when developing more potent health practices. When you value the opportunities that life offers with each new day, an experience like cancer helps you recognize the worth of having more time to be more appreciative of all the things often taken for granted, like hugs from your children, watching them explore and discover, and reminiscing and laughing with a spouse. Even going to work can be enjoyable. Oops, did I go too far?

Relationships

One's attitude influences relationships too. Some people can cheer up a whole room when they enter it, while others do so by leaving it. It is incredible to me how one person's negative energy can drain the life out of others. Try being around a chronic complainer, critic, or disagreeable person, even briefly, and you'll experience a shift in mood. When my spirit is not upbeat, usually I'm experiencing fatigue, and my thoughts focus on the negative. Sometimes, it is because I'm not feeling well or am allowing others' negative inputs to influence my mood. Change one of these variables by focusing on a positive aspect and watch energy increase and relationships begin to thrive.

To develop a more positive approach to life, start simply. It can be as easy as avoiding the "downer Debbies and Dougies" of the world, but this can also be complicated. Unfortunately, too many times, close friends or, worse, our family members pollute our minds. The worst ones try to outdo you by letting everyone know how much worse their life is than other people's. They are so proud of their misery that they must share it with anyone willing to listen. Like there is a reward for the one living the most miserable life, they have to outdo others by telling a bigger sob story than anyone else. If you cannot avoid these individuals, do your best to change the subject to something else. In the beginning, make it something benign. "Hey, did you watch the game last night?" Or maybe compliment them or recall a humorous incident. If nothing comes to mind, choose a general subject, such as how good the weather has been. Try to shift the conversation from negative to neutral, then with time, a more positive, even inspiring one.

There are those people who cheer us up when we are around them. Interact with people who bring energy to your life; spend a limited time with those who are energy/life draining. If you find yourself in an unavoidable situation, try to control the energy of a conversation—interject positive and empowering thoughts, ideas, and possibilities in a conversation when possible. When necessary, recognize a perceived negative incident as a learning opportunity; not as an outcome but as a beginning, to build and improve a function or responsibility.

If you dislike a particular situation or task, be it at work or personally, investigate why it is that way. There could be a valid rationale behind a specific action. If there is an improved alternative, try it or present it to others; acquire some critical evaluation, pros, and cons, and then reconsider and decide what is prudent before acting.

It is said, "We become like the people we surround ourselves with." Examining this statement relative to people I know, evidence supports it. For a recovering person from any addiction, it is tough to expect to stay sober if they surround themselves with old friends who encourage or embrace their previous lifestyle. There are many incidences where removing a person from a hostile environment to a more positive, supportive one changes that individual for the better.

A movie from my youth, starring comic actors Eddie Murphy and Dan Akroyd, called *Trading Places*, plays on this theme. In it, a homeless man, Eddie Murphy, was taken off the street by two financially successful brothers, adopted into a lifestyle, and taught the skills to become wealthy, while his counterpart, Dan Akroyd, was removed from a rich environment to live like a pauper. Each finds themselves in a role reversal and living the lifestyle of their environment. Not only can this occur in Hollywood, but it can also be true in life. Change the setting and you can influence the personality.

How one copes with the reality of cancer will influence the quality of the time ahead. Surrounding yourself with positive people will affect the experience of each new day. I'm not saying to associate with or listen to only people who offer ridiculous platitudes or condemn you for having moments of feeling badly physically and emotionally. However, that may be better than an individual who brings nothing more than pity. It would help if you had people who appreciate what you are going through and avoid those who offer only sympathy. If you assist one on this journey, be supportive while offering positive stimulation with valuable foods, physical activity, and encouraging words.

Something you can do for yourself to help with stress and anxiety is to get involved in doing things, contributing to people and causes, or finding projects that need attention. For example, with the help of a professional and family, we remade my mother's landscaping. As a result, I was moving my thoughts away from excessive worrying about the future and more about the present, while also giving me feelings of satisfaction by helping someone else.

Seeking support from friends, family, medical personnel, and groups became a valuable way for me to relieve some of the anxieties from the lack of information. Becoming withdrawn will only worsen your concerns and aids no one, especially the patient. Referring to what I said earlier about the people you surround yourself with, be selective of who you allow into your inner circle, including support groups. Some support groups were nothing more than pity parties—too many negative vibes. As worthwhile as it is to know others understand the experience of cancer, there must be a significant emphasis on taking practical steps towards dealing with the disease emotionally and physically, not just the negative consequences; not to be in a state of denial but rather one of finding positive inputs valuable to your journey.

The influence of affirming people and groups, accepting your condition, then seeking information on what you can do personally, and acting on it, makes you a problem solver. Become self-empowering. You are being led to the fighting spirit needed to gain an edge and prevail over the whole cancer experience. Know that punishing yourself or self-blame benefits no one, especially you, and can only weaken your resolve to face the challenges ahead. Often, the emotional pain that we experience comes from within. Our choices, perceptions of life, and self-talk all shape how we experience any event, including an illness like cancer. How you grapple with the ordeal will influence your quality of life. When you create more affirming and productive, self-directed methods and beliefs, you will be introduced to the more powerful person you can be.

Support groups can be a valuable coping tool. But be very careful with which ones you become involved. Expressing emotions can be a good stress release. The issue with groups is that they seem to be more about supporting you in misery than helping you deal with cancer in the most effective ways possible. Just giving you a shoulder to cry on won't increase your odds of beating cancer. I lasted through only two meetings of hearing life stories, some repeated from the previous gathering. I am more interested in what I can do with better communication skills with my doctor and where to get helpful information and strategies to win the battle for my life. Now you have my attention when you share what you've learned and how it served you. If you choose to participate in a support group, studies indicate the most valuable ones promote strategies you can implement, like coping skills, lifestyle adaptations, and relaxation strategies.

A simple step is to stay connected and restore and develop social relationships. **HARVARD WOMEN'S HEALTH** periodical says quality social relationships can reduce stress and stress-inducing hormones, thereby enhancing the immune system's functions. Social activity can range from positive, friendly connections, to supporting others. Here is the exciting part: Regardless of whether you are the giver or the receiver of such interactions, both parties will experience life-enhancing benefits. The advantage of this health-enhancing step of becoming involved with others is that it's easy and has many options and low cost. A network of quality, supportive relationships is a good starting point for creating a positive, mindful, calm focal point.

Create and build relationships with people through small acts of kindness. Release the need to be judgmental towards others and especially yourself. There are enough critics to go around; there is no need for another, and you are probably the most critical of yourself and unaware of it. Remember the golden rule: "Do unto others as you would like to be done unto." You can only do for others what you are willing to do for yourself.

Words Matter

Much of the emphasis on health focuses on staying active and what we feed our tummies, which are critical to physical and mental well-being. But how about what we provide our minds by what we read and listen to, our viewing habits, and what has become an incredible influencer, social media?

I'll go out on a limb and say that a few of us have not been negatively affected by someone or something posted online. It is usually a matter of comparing ourselves and our lives to those people showing all the incredibly positive things happening in their lives, which is good. But in the same vein as the scene with the wizard from the Wizard of Oz at the Emerald City, pay no attention to social media. If you could pull back the curtain, it becomes apparent that no one is posting their failures.

However, some find it necessary to share their victimhood publicly by proclaiming to the world the misery in their life. I wonder whether they seek sympathy or want attention. Yet, I am convinced that it is not benefiting them and their health. On the contrary, those who live life from the standpoint of misery are subject to elevated stress levels, leading to adverse mental and physical health consequences. Whatever you focus on, you find more of it, positive or negative.

Another area to work on is your language. I'm not referring to spewing foul words out of your mouth. However, these types of comments could be more inspiring by simply finding better expressions for the events that most of us do regularly, like going to work or school, or doing tasks, "honey do's" around the house, or any other things many of us perform daily. Changing how we choose to express duties typical to many people can transform how we approach life.

Psychologist Bea, of the **Cleveland Clinic,** says, "...our brain responds very powerfully to the way we use language when we talk and in the way we use language in our thoughts." Using different words like "I get to..." instead of "I have to..." can change a burden into an opportunity. Enthusiasm accompanies opportunity because we view things as a benefit.

Instead of dreading the idea of a change in diet and habits as denying yourself the little pleasures you may have assigned to junk food or a no-effort sedentary lifestyle, choose to adopt ideas such as, "Today is the first day of my new healthy life, filled with energy and opportunities to enjoy." How you talk to yourself and others can affect your behavior. Trash talking about bad habits by you and others threatens your self-esteem. An upbeat, self-affirming personal communication style opens our minds to be more receptive to new healthy ideas.

Research published in **Proceedings of the National Academies of Science** indicated that crucial brain areas are activated when a person receives self-affirming information regarding health advice. Furthermore, these levels remain for weeks after the initial observation. In contrast, health advice given negatively showed lower brain activity levels and a continued sedentary lifestyle.

Vanessa Patrick and her research team considered a change in how we phrase a thought or sentence and its effect on one's actions. They found that simply changing a single word can increase the motivation center, making us more likely to stay focused on the desired outcome.

For example, instead of saying, "I can't do...," choose the words, "I don't do...." This simple change shifts motivational control from external to internal. When motivated from within, we are more likely to stay focused on what we want in the long run. Imagine a healthier lifestyle being born from, "I don't eat junk food. I'm choosing to eat more vegetables, fruits, berries, and other nutritious foods." Sometimes, significant shifts in life start with a simple step taken today, like adopting words that put you in control. It is worth considering as you move toward a more positive way of living.

Embracing a constructive modification of attitude towards new healthful habits can motivate us to stick to it while increasing happiness. Positivity is a powerful way to create change in life. Starting simply by taking on new words, phrases, and thoughts, inclined to inspire action and appreciate the benefits of this conversion, may be the catalyst needed for more livelihood. When viewing the idea of something, or someone for that matter, as a burden, the brain processes it as a threat to you, your freedom, livelihood, and so on, making it less likely you will incorporate positive changes into your life. Reframing these moments as challenges presents us with opportunities that arouse a desire to succeed at a life test and remove the threat. Think about it: Would you rather be presented with a threat or a challenge? Though cancer threatened my family and me, I elected to take it on as a challenge by not letting cancer win or beat me. I did this by changing my diet, lifestyle, and attitude, defining winning as not allowing cancer to have my liveliness by living, and appreciating the present moment and not just succumbing to the ravaging effects it can cause.

Crazy as it may seem, simply referring to cancer in other terms can be helpful. According to breast cancer specialist **Laura Esserman, MD**, at the **University of California, San Francisco**, "cancer" arouses thoughts of a need to hurry. Yet, this may not be the case. Instead, she says, "Patients rush into treatments that might have long-term negative consequences." Better, more informed decisions are possible when there doesn't exist the feeling of rushing into medical therapies, leading to healthier choices. By referring to cancer as lesions on an organ's linings, Dr. Esserman and her team deemphasized it as an aggressive killer to an affliction with treatment options. Refocusing may stop an unnecessary operation, like a radical mastectomy when a lumpectomy is a reasonable choice. Evaluating the possibilities is what is valuable. Steps can include second, third, or how many opinions it may take from other doctors to allow you to feel confident entrusting your health to them, aiding you in making smarter, healthier, more informed decisions.

Dr. Brennan, one of my oncologists and who diagnosed multiple myeloma, referred to "lesions" on several of my skeletal regions, relaxing a sense of urgency that comes when we often hear the words, "You have cancer." This enabled me to investigate possible therapies I could engage in while medical personnel evaluated their preferences, benefits, and consequences of their choice of treatments. It gave me some peace of mind that death wasn't imminent, allowing the medical team, and me, time to respond positively to the diagnosis while believing my best interests were being considered.

There is emerging psychotherapy around focusing on little tweaks to how we talk. It includes using our internal communications to empower us when we find ourselves in tough times like cancer. Internal communication involves self-talk, imagination, feelings, and the emotions they generate. For example, a positive perspective can persuade us to become increasingly thankful. Cultivating an "attitude of gratitude" encourages us to expand positive communications within us, encouraging productive behaviors. On the other hand, a negative view of life tends to be defeating by its nature. An adverse focus on your life cultivates a cycle of negativism, increasing fearful thoughts and hindering the possibility of becoming your desired person.

The brain's emotional centers are influenced by how we define our state. When it comes to anxiety and excitement, both these emotions activate the same area of the brain in the prefrontal cortex. Researcher Alison Brooks has demonstrated that choosing a more positive, purposeful word over a negative one can help overcome anxiety and enhance performance. Her simple linguistic strategy is to restate feelings of anxiety as ones of excitement. Instead of focusing on anxiousness, reframe it as the emotion of excitement. Tell yourself and others how excited you are to be able to ____ (reference whatever you tend to be hostile towards). In addition to reducing anxiety, we tend to perform at a higher level when we are excited.

It all started with the words I chose. Instead of, "Why did this happen to me?" I'm learning to try, "How can I use this to...?" Incorporating better questions into my internal communication has become empowering. I no longer throw up my hands and think I can do nothing about an individual occurrence. Instead, I've learned there is always something I can do. It may be as simple as, "What did that experience teach me?" Applying this principle during the cancer years empowered me to look for ways to contribute to my well-being. I did this through a better diet, adding nutritionally-packed, natural immune-boosting plants and spices, finding more quiet time, and feeding my mind with the positive psychology of what is possible. The possibility thinker accepts an outcome as an experience to grow forward and shape a better response to future challenges.

Releasing negative talk, whether directed at yourself or others, can be difficult. To assist in being more affirming, look to your core values. Are they positive or lean toward the negative? They are often rooted in experiences perceived to be positive and negative. Either way, there is purpose in those things that matter most to us—these core values center on seeking pleasure and avoiding what we perceive as threatening. Averting the need to assign blame to a person or event removes what is considered a risk. There is no reason to blame. Accepting each outcome as only a learning opportunity, preparing us for the future, enables us to release the negative while empowering us by focusing on the positive learning aspects of events, others, and ourselves.

The Voice Within

A habit ripe for review is your self-talk. These words may be the most destructive or constructive dialogue you'll ever have. So what conversations are you having with that little voice inside? The effect may not be so little. To alter a saying I've heard, change your words, change your mindset, change your habits—change your life.

STANFORD REPORTS, a periodical of **STANFORD UNIVERSITY** that describes their mission as helping humans thrive, published an interview with Dr. Jacob Towery, an adjunct clinical instructor in the department of psychiatry. First, he states that one's mindset is the filter through which we perceive life and develop our expectations. An example is, "...believe that becoming sick with cancer would be catastrophic or that going on a diet would be challenging and depriving." These assumptions lead to worst-case scenario thinking. The inner voice and conscious and unconscious beliefs make up one's mindset. It can be either valuable or misguided, with feelings of guilt, inadequacy, sadness, and anxiety developing from false negative beliefs of oneself.

Dr. Towery reveals that mindset influences even physiology, referencing studies on the placebo effects and medications. Results show a positive outcome of as high as 40 percent in some studies, just from taking a sugar pill thought to be an effective medication by the patient. He promises that mindset is changeable. If you have an attitude of growth and are willing to take the steps necessary to do it, this will spur an increase in happiness and health.

We often discount the power of the mind-body connection. Self-talk matters because it affects confidence, feelings (beneficial or harmful), and health, and may limit the willingness to act toward more favorable outcomes. The little voice within leads both the victor and the victim; depending on the channel you choose to tune into, giving it validation becomes your truth, thereby determining the quality of your life.

Statements that use the word "I," such as, "I feel terrific!" assign ownership to a trait, desirable or unfavorable. Be careful with what words you adopt to fill in the blank. Be sure to choose empowering thoughts, ideas, and words that provoke positive feelings, while avoiding the ones that promote emotions of defeat. While battling cancer, for example, as I drifted to sleep each night, I would repeat to myself, "I am healthy," to convince the subconscious to wake up my bodily systems to get to work, helping me to create a healthy consciousness. Positive self-talk is not a substitute for positive actions but a compliment to your efforts to achieve a goal, health in this case.

Be conscious of the words you choose in all conversations, internal and with others. There is power in them, and you want them to be constructive, not destructive. Building an empowering mindset begins with believing that you can handle it, whatever that "it" may be, regardless of the outcome. And that belief can be shaped by words, spoken and unspoken, so watch your language. When drifting into discouraging thoughts, change direction simply by doing something you enjoy, especially if it involves physical movement and is done with someone that brings joy to the moment. You are tougher than you know and are capable of meeting your challenges; self-talk is an excellent place to start.

Hope

A doctor once told me, "Don't get your hopes up." Sorry doc, I did anyway. I believe hope is what drives us to try and improve our predicament. The boundaries we set for ourselves become our limits. In the Bible, the book of Proverbs tells us, "Hope deferred makes a heart sick." Instead, discover a burning hope from the emotional heart to push you to endure more than possible. The greater our belief that what we do matters, the more likely we will act empoweringly. We are limited only by the size of our hope.

Many may say that I am only spreading false hope. Following science or medicine will decide the best outcome. Let me clarify. I am not trying to have you turn your back on any corrective measures that medical knowledge deems appropriate. What I am highlighting is what you already know. Without going all in, the result is limited. To conquer any great challenge, you must be willing to go above and beyond "good enough." Modifying a quote from the late Henry Ford,

"Whether you believe what you do matters or believe it doesn't, you're right," if for no other reason except that hope is an attitude of determination not to let a cancer condition take your emotional soul. To be as healthy as you can be, you must become a better version of yourself mentally, physically, and emotionally.

The Covington, Kentucky, Diocesan Catholic Children's Home (DCCH) is a local organization that assists families and challenged youth in their developmental years. I've had a past relationship with it as a volunteer. "Dean," as portrayed in one of the home's publications, was described as a "brave young man" who became a resident. Mr. Miller was the first person he met at DCCH, and through the years, he became a significant guide to Dean. I will share some excerpts from a poem he wrote called **HOPE**. His relationship with his mentor, Mr. Miller, who has since passed, inspired Dean to write it.

"Hope is something that makes us thrive.
Yes, hope is what keeps us alive."
"Let our hope guide us in the right direction."
"Hope makes us persistent, gives us resistance,
and it helps carry us the distance."
"It's the things that we hope for, that show who we are."

It's essential to have an optimistic hope for the best possible outcome. Yet, it may be hopeless without believing in your ability to influence the journey. Making a practical shift in your diet, lifestyle, environment, and spirit is equally valuable to a successful outcome as modern medicine, while implementing changes in these areas of your life includes increasing hope with a positive mental attitude, and stress management with mindfulness and meditation. Each helps build the body's defenses for a more robust response to cancer. It leads to a more constructive response than one of helplessness.

We must live with the belief that what we do can make a difference. Our circumstances are not our destiny. What has happened to you does not define what can happen or what you can accomplish. It's never too late to start your campaign of winning over cancer, understanding that it is a process, and it is a combination of your actions, physical and mental, that is going to make a difference. Open your mind to the possibility of conquering cancer and embrace the mindset of not letting cancer have your spirit.

Believing that you can be victorious may start with redefining how you view cancer. As with any fear in all areas of life, our angst may be attributable to stories we've heard. These depictions of unpleasantness and despair may arise from others we know who have had the disease, as I mentioned with the older gentleman who believes that cancer treatments would make him feel miserable. So, initially, he chose not to be treated, being unaware of medications available to counteract some of those experiences. Maybe a lack of knowledge and understanding of the treatments or information given to you by medical professionals is void of options or possibilities.

Purpose

Think of anything you are successful at doing in your life, and you'll find crucial personal characteristics you first employed: the desire to do it and the belief you could do it. The more you establish the desire to thrive in your heart, the greater your commitment to the process will lead to better results. The most beneficial outcomes in all areas of life come from being all in. Embodying the concept of personal responsibility for your health opens the potentiality and synergies of mind, body, spirit, and emotions with positive expectations. Your greater devotion leads to more empowering beliefs, allowing for the best possible results.

The cancer experience is challenging for the family, friends, and patient. In addition to being physically draining, treatments are emotionally and mentally exhausting. Add to that, anxiety and hopelessness; now you have a recipe for immune suppression and cancer progression. Together they reduce the capacity of the body to heal. Lifestyle adaptation is necessary to transform your condition favorably.

It can be helpful motivation to find purpose in your affliction. I found it beneficial to continually ask myself, "How can I use this for constructive change?" and "Can my journey be of value to others?" These questions came to me when I prayed and talked with God about what my family would do without me. During this moment, I got a sense of creating a fresh perspective, that my attitudes and efforts were in my control. It was up to me to step up and resolve to be the best me I could be.

Along with defining meaning, I also daydreamed of a positive, happy future for myself and my family, creating a more positive emotional experience. Together, they produce a unique harmony that can be transformative. An optimistic outlook is valuable to achieving a better state of mind. With it, changing your habits, essential to a desirable outcome, becomes increasingly more accessible. In addition, they boost the body's natural healing abilities while enhancing the immune system.

Researchers have established that those who win over cancer take an integrative approach—seeking unique techniques and standard conventional therapies. Patients can take control of their health by looking beyond traditional medicine and operating more intuitively. When we feel in control, we enjoy a greater sense of peace. Your mindset, your beliefs, and your actions are essential. Combined, they shape your outcome.

These will help to strengthen you physically. When the body feels more robust, we are encouraged to fight onward and beyond what we may have thought was possible. Reject the disease's psychological hold on you by embracing life through these physically and emotionally demanding times. Keep living. Looking forward to each day focused on what you can do while not worrying about what others say is impossible. If you ever saw the movie *Angels in the Outfield,* one little boy would respond," Could happen," as it related to crazy possibilities. Make "could happen" your new mantra on life's possibilities.

Please, whatever you do, do not play the blame game, especially with yourself. Steer away from the things that create emotional distress, as it will likely lead to more negative feelings. Anxiety in life promotes inflammatory ammunition for growth and the spread of tumors. Instead, focus on dealing with the disease by obtaining the best possible treatments, personally contributing to lifestyle changes, and being committed to living your best possible life. It begins with a belief in the achievement of restoring well-being.

My purpose in this area is to increase awareness that if you think because your friend Fred died from cancer, and now you have it, you're doomed, or it runs in the family, this is not true. After many years of being cancer free, it was conveyed to me by one of my oncologists to keep doing what I was doing, because they did not expect me to make it. My efforts began with me believing that I could influence the experience. Other people's results do not have to equal mine; I am not a statistic, and neither are you.

Genetic mutation carriers have an increased risk of experiencing a type of cancer, but not everyone**.** David Michael Euhus, M.D., **Professor of Surgery** at **John Hopkins Medicine**, with expertise in breast cancer, recommends regular testing and working with your doctor to take preventative steps to lower the risk, if you have the mutation of the BRACA genes. In addition, positive living through a healthy diet, including what you feed your mind and other wholesome habits, like improving lifestyle and diet, is a part of protective strategies.

Finding active and inactive ways to manage the psychological burdens each day is essential to a positive response to dealing with cancer disease. Proper rest, a more powerful diet, and a positive psychological approach are all necessary to meet and beat the challenges of the disease, as it is with any life test.

Chapter 13

What Now?

"The way to get started is to quit talking and begin doing."
– Walt Disney

Does it make a difference to incorporate many aspects as possible steps to overcome cancer's grip on you? Some say, "It's a waste of time and money." However, changing your lifestyle, exercising, and increasing the fruits and vegetables in your diet, and adding supplements, will help you feel better and have increased energy. These areas alone will empower you to take the necessary steps and not give up the fight.

The Iron Man Triathlon is a race involving three separate legs: a 2.4-mile swim, a 112-mile bicycle ride, and a 26.2-mile run. I don't know about you, but this would take me about a week to complete in good physical condition. The contestants do it in hours. Let's say you were going to participate in this incredibly challenging race. Would you show up unprepared or conditioned? Whether you are ready or not, it takes commitment and focus, and you must dedicate yourself to the desired outcome. If you aren't mentally primed, you will run out of whatever it takes to see it through.

The cancer experience is like a triathlon. The initial phase is when medical science attacks cancer with chemical therapies and radiation. But whether this destroys the cancer or not, you have just started, and the journey of winning over cancer continues. The treatments now damage your body, and it needs reconstruction. But just any rebuilding won't do. First, restoring your physical self with new substantial cells is necessary. It begins with adopting new dietary habits; next is the marathon of sticking with the lifestyle changes you have created.

New habits of diet, stress relief, exercise, mindfulness, and other unique patterns are critical to a new you. Once the body is free of these rogue cells, the most immediate action you can take is to provide nutritional resources to chemically change and balance the biome called the body. This is to shift the progress of the disease, and also for the marathon of life for a prolonged, better-quality of life, long-term remission, and optimal health.

An integrative approach to dealing with any physical disease equally applies to psychological challenges, whether it is cancer or life stressors. It doesn't limit your options; it increases them. The doctors do their part, but with integrative medicine, you can implement the new lifestyle or the changes necessary to have a life over cancer. It is a multi-dimensional method that requires a spirit of desire for living, the strength to discipline yourself to do whatever it takes, and the courage to continue the battle against the odds. To move a mountain requires lifting many rocks, mostly one at a time.

One of the pioneers in integrative oncology I mentioned earlier, is Doctor Keith Block, the founder of **The Block Center for Integrative Cancer Treatment** in Chicago, Illinois. His center was a part of my initial efforts and investigation into cancer. His book, *Life Over Cancer*, was one of my sources for developing a better approach to winning my crusade to beat the odds. In searching for how to be a victor and not a victim, I learned that an integrative approach was the best chance of winning.

Contrary to the information publicly available, modern pharmacology has not found a cure for cancer or most of the chronic disease we humans are dealing with today—only ways to control the affliction. To beat any disease, such as type 2 diabetes, hypertension, or cancer, it takes an active approach on the part of the individual. Otherwise, it will be temporary. Integrating nutrition, exercise, improved mental outlooks, and a revised lifestyle are all important to include in whatever defined treatments your healthcare providers are using to combat a disease.

For example, a recent study of 50 lung cancer patients, who wore pedometers to count their steps, found those who were the least active were also most likely to have the least desirable outcome. Fifty percent of those with the lowest number of steps required hospitalization while being treated, and 55 percent of those patients died within 18 months. In comparison, only nine percent of the more active participants required hospitalization during treatments. Fewer than 25 percent of them died during the study.

Being resolute in your activity levels while receiving your treatments is crucial. Those patients in this study who walked less during treatments were at a higher risk of being hospitalized. As I've indicated, exercise is essential. Something as simple as walking can make a difference.

While striving to beat acute myeloid leukemia, I was hooked up to chemotherapy 24 hours a day for seven days, twice. I required hospitalization during treatments. After visiting hours, when only a diminished staff occupied the hallways, I would walk, rolling my tower of chemo and tubes through the halls to stay as active as possible. Even after my transplants at the Mayo Clinic, my caregiver and I would walk to and from doctors' appointments in the winter cold and on a treadmill at night. As the weather improved, I was there from winter into early summer; we began to ride bikes on the beautiful trails around the City of Rochester, Minnesota. Not only was this physically beneficial, but being outside was also good psychologically. I'm not sure what came first; feeling good physically, so I was active; or being involved, which helped me feel better in many aspects, including increased appetite.

Through epigenetics studies, science has learned that our health is influenced by more than our genes. Cancer, for instance, starts from exposure to environmental conditions, ranging from radiation, both what is natural from the sun or artificial, and toxic compounds found in the air we breathe, the water we drink, the food we eat, and chronic stress. These disrupt standard physiological mechanisms within our bodies, creating cell mutations by altering their DNA.

You will enhance the medically accepted treatments by including better quality nutrition, exercise, attentiveness to your mindset, and affirmative lifestyle changes. To be and stay cancer-free requires more than just removing or destroying malignant cells through medical therapeutics. There is an ongoing battle that takes place daily within the body to eliminate mutant and damaged cells. Yet, there are times when the body becomes overwhelmed, and the body's natural defenses are unable to kill off abnormal cells.

This book aims to provide information that your oncology/hematology team may not offer, and to express what I've learned and applied in my life to beat cancer and stay cancer-free, not to be disparaging about the medical community. All the ones I've met are knowledgeable and well-educated and are interested in your health as they understand it. Yet, in much medical training, less than 1% of the educational process is on the valuable subject of nutrition, even though a significant part of the immune system is the digestive tract. An unhealthy gut can often be created by poor eating habits, leading to many chronic illnesses.

Improving the outcome of your experience is possible by employing a "wholistic" approach to care, as described earlier. The results I have enjoyed, and those of other victors, speak to the value of an integrative treatment program. You, as the patient, need to take control of your destiny by first asking questions of your oncologist and their team members. Be careful what you accept from them as absolute truth.

Lack of information among some medical professionals leads to thinking, "If it were true, they would teach it in med-school," creating among some in medicine an attitude of, "If it doesn't come in a pill, an injectable, or from a laboratory, then it's not worth considering as a viable treatment or benefit." "Follow the science" is a common declaration. If one defines science as knowledge gained by observation, studying, and asking questions, accordingly, then there are many overlooked possibilities in areas of medicine. Challenging accepted practices, opinions, and principles is how we gain advances in science, medicine, and all areas of life. Therefore, all the information I have reported may be considered science; not my opinion but knowledge gained and recorded through observations in laboratory experiments by professionals in their fields of study and through real-life examples. I am acting as a reporter for such information.

Some strict conventional medicine practitioners may tell you there is no supporting evidence for anything included in this book. If their experience focuses on only applying their medical school training received in the United States, I understand that view. But there are increasingly more studies from research at major universities and laboratories, in and outside the U.S., providing new realms of information. These investigations into functional approaches, integrated with conventional treatments, offer various possibilities for an improved experience when dealing with chronic diseases ranging from dementia to cancer. It may be better to consider holistic medicine to be "wholistic." This approach involves the whole person, diet, lifestyle, exercise, mental state, and development. After all, they are all health care. A growing number of conventionally educated physicians are open to new ideas and additional possibilities available for their patients.

I am intimately familiar with a case of a man with myelodysplastic syndrome (MDS), preleukemia, whose doctors choose not to treat him because of his age. They even ignored his questions for almost a year about his condition by acting as if they were trying to determine what was ailing him. Family and friends established his disorder through their research, later confirmed by his doctor. It appears as if the doctor(s) were choosing his outcome for him; this is wrong in so many ways.

After an unrelated additional medical condition pushed his MDS to acute myeloid leukemia, the doctor's prognosis jumped to dire. I was present when this family, whose father was in his 70s, was asking questions of the doctor about the options available. I was astonished when the doctor said, "Mister _______, nothing can be done. You have a lovely family; why don't you just go home and wait until it's over." Excuse me, but who made him the arbiter of life? Obviously, this doctor flunked or skipped the classes on bedside manners—time to find another doctor, ASAP.

His new doctor's first comment was that the prognosis was probably correct unless he was willing to fight. He didn't promise anything to the family except that by following an integrative approach, he could gain extended time with his family. Unfortunately, four days later, he died from lack of treatment related to his condition, but not specifically because of the disease. The second doctor believes, given the proper care in the beginning, this man would have had additional years with his family. It is crucial to do all you can do, as soon as you can do it, for the most significant possibility of winning, including not settling for one doctor's opinion, especially when it appears that their only interest is in treating the disease more than the person who has it.

Doing your part begins with taking steps to change or adjust your lifestyle. One of the most effective things I did was to evaluate my diet. Through my investigation into how food can influence our body, I learned that plants contain an array of phytonutrients that, when consumed regularly, can contribute to a change in our body's chemistry.

As you know, a positive lifestyle is more than just the food we eat. It includes exercise, stress reduction, proper rest, and what we feed our minds. When combined, these lifestyle adjustments can help change the biochemistry within us that has supported cancer development and propagation and is valid for other chronic diseases we may acquire over time. Work with your integrative physician to design an individual plan that can be a basis for enhanced therapies, to be the difference that matters prospectively.

There are thousands of reports on cancer cures through natural means. Though I have not validated them, these are credible accounts of individuals who follow a strict organic plant diet, including juicing, supplementation, and additional holistic treatments. This can possibly be attributed to the anti-inflammatory, antioxidant, and adverse cancer properties found naturally in plants. This approach, mostly involving oversight by a skilled medical practitioner, is designed around care for all aspects of the patient, not just centered around one issue.

Often, these patient's diagnosis is that their disease has progressed so far that conventional medical care offers little hope. But the patient had hope—a personal intent for living, and they were prepared to do whatever it took to see their purpose fulfilled. It is a powerful mechanism, purpose. It keeps us believing in our dreams and desires, pulling us toward our future with a willingness to bear considerable sacrifices and discomfort to bring it into fruition. These are the people who will not take NO or CAN'T as final. They search to find a way where others said there is no way.

I am not saying to go it alone. The most prudent advice is to combine natural means with current medical treatments, an integrative approach, to achieve the best possible results. Scientific research shows that the results are greatly enhanced through the combination of wholesome and conventional methods. Be suspect of any medical practitioners who disqualify your personal efforts to beat the disease. A passion for living has tremendous power beyond what science understands. Without a drive to do whatever it takes, your resolution to succeed becomes narrow. Through my experience with "one option" types of people, in any area of health care, a majority of them know little about nutrition, powerful phytochemicals, and possible remedies or benefits outside the traditional Western approach to medicine.

Research would confirm that Western medicine is incredibly successful at dealing with acute challenges. It possesses some of the most intelligent and skilled individuals in their fields. However, I have learned that being highly educated does not always translate to mean well rounded knowledge or being fully informed. Sometimes, the more education one has, it seems to lend itself to an attitude of smugness by some, toward possibilities and alternatives to explore and/or include things that do not fit the conventional narrative.

There is a story I love that is a reminder of not dismissing what may seem too elementary. If you've heard it, then this is a good reminder. If not, it will provide a little chuckle while providing the wisdom of considering simple solutions. A large truck and its driver were in a predicament. The truck was stuck under an overpass and was unable to move forward or back. Authorities had shown up on the scene and many minds were deliberating on the best solution to the problem, with no real consensus on how to solve it. A little boy who had been watching and listening to the conversations with curiosity, approached one of the investigative experts and said, "Hey, mister, why don't you just let the air out of the tires." There was laughter at the foolish idea of a naive mind. After more deliberation and no viable solution, the tow truck driver, who had shown up late at the spectacle, reviewed the situation and offered, "If we deflate the tires, I can pull the truck clear. I have an air compressor on the tow truck, so I can then re-inflate the tires." It was successful.

Whether the story is from an actual incident or not, I'm not sure. But it brings to light that sometimes, simple actions make the difference. Also, occasionally the intelligent mind overlooks the innocent possibilities available because it is difficult to believe in the simple as being effective. Being healthy can be that way. The remedy may be as easy as a lifestyle adjustment, better choices of food and drink, walking regularly, and some mental downtime. These self empowering actions are so incredibly simple and known to be beneficial, yet there are 1001 excuses as to why they are not followed. Introducing prospective advantages often leads to fresh thinking and unique possibilities in all areas of life. But you have to put them to work. Knowledge not applied is worthless.

Healthy

I once heard a statement credited to writer and poet Maya Angelou, "Be careful when a naked man offers you his shirt." Initially, that brings a little giggle, but when I thought about it, I realize that it applies to so many areas of life when we are looking for some type of insight or guidance on what to do next. Too many times, we ask for advice from someone who has no more or even less experience in a given area than we do. This seems to be more common when it comes to relationships and politics. I hope I have convinced you that I am not that naked man offering you a shirt. But I have bared it all to you, in an effort to get you more engaged in the outcome of your health.

Your lifestyle is an integral part to your recovery and staying healthy. If you have been sedentary most of your adult life or most recently, it's time to change. Exercise does many things to the body. One is that it stresses it in a positive way. Exposure to intervals of positive physical stress can be of value because it helps prepare the body for other types of stress that may be detrimental to your health. Crazy as it sounds, it also can help release mental and emotional tension. Another is that the movement of muscles acts as a pump to keep fluid moving through the lymph system, as a part of the detoxification process of the body.

Also, the food that we consume can either be empty calories or high-octane ones. You need valuable nutrients along with energy to recover from the bombardment of toxins we are continually exposed to, including from chemotherapy and radiation. Every day, there are toxins that accompany the foods we consume in the form of pesticides, products we use, and the air we breathe. For instance, there are chemicals like benzene, a cancer-causing agent, from the vapors we inhale when we add gas to our cars.

Earlier, I referred to the experience of dealing with cancer as a journey, because it is exactly that. If you are diagnosed with any chronic disease, especially cancer, a shot or pill isn't going to cure it. Nor is a single round of chemo or radiation treatments. Hence, it is a chronic disease.

The way you are going to become a victor over cancer is to decide to do all you can do.

The song "Stumble On," by the rock group Wayback, is about addiction, recovery, and the weight of the challenges faced to overcome it, tough as it may be. This is not unique to an addiction. It is a way of life for all. From the time we begin life on this Earth, we are exploring and conquering bits and pieces of a world. Each stride forward exposes us to stumbling blocks. Those things that trip us can become foundational blocks to build our future. Think about a child learning to walk. To continue with an attitude and determination, can enable us to experience life more fully.

Each day offers experiences, building blocks of opportunities, that can be the foundation for greater things. Under the weight of failures, setbacks, and challenges, we "stumble on" towards a feeling that we won the day, or we experienced setbacks. Some days, there will be big wins, but the majority will be mini ones. When dealing with cancer, for instance, "I went for a walk today," or "I ate and kept the food down," and "I felt better today" seem like little nothings to bystanders, but for the patient, it can be a big deal. There are no minor victories. Count each win as a building block towards your ultimate definition of victory.

Reflect back on those moments when you were pursuing a goal, either as a child or adult—maybe a top grade in school, making a sports team, riding a bike, the affection of a mate—anything that you think of as winning. Then it felt like one more obstacle was dropped in front you, blocking the path to a goal. It may have tripped you, but then you used it as a building block for a stronger foundation for your desired outcome. With the little adjustments, you steered towards the destination.

The type of person reading this book is most likely a believer in changing their life by taking charge of the things they can control: attitude, effort, habits, diet, and so on. If so, then you have probably heard that an airplane and its pilot are continuously making minor adjustments to make it to the destination. Wind, weather, turbulence, magnetic variations, and a number of other forces make this necessary. This is the analogy for life. Daily, there are adjustments that need to be made to keep us on course. As long as we make them, we'll arrive where we intended to go. If you don't change bad habits, you will be at the mercy of outside forces. Keep doin' whatcha doin', and ya keep gett'n whatcha gett'n. It is the little changes that can lead to the big difference.

I use the word victor instead of survivor because, for me, saying, "I'm a survivor" denotes that I am still in the state of victimhood. But as a victor, I have won. I am victorious in my cause to not let a life of possibilities be taken from me. Let me decide when it is finished, even if it is just in a state of mind.

I'm reminded of the scene in the movie *Braveheart*, when Mel Gibson's character William Wallace is about to be executed. In a moment of total defiance, he yells out, "FREEDOM!" That is what being a victor is to me—the freedom to choose a course of action and pursue it with passion—not denying one has cancer or any other life event that has set you back, but to strive forward towards living the best you can be in the moment. Like the apostle Paul wrote when on death row, "Forgetting those things that lie in the past, I press forward."

My Swan Song

It took me awhile to write this book for multiple reasons. First, I wanted my life without cancer to be a testament to the guidance that I offer in this book. My doctors and I believe I am doing something right. Next, it took awhile to review and validate the information as reliable. I enjoy a giggle every now and again when I'm traveling on an airplane out of uniform. It's usually a unique situation and the person near me is voicing their inaccurate and incomplete expertise on the plane or flying. My attempt was for that not to be me, as related to health. Finally, this is my first attempt at writing anything other than required college papers, and a couple of magazine articles, expressing myself takes time. Hence, the writing style is a less established book style and more of a conversational mode of expression.

Admittedly, I didn't know what I was in for when I started down this path of trying to convey valuable, effective information in an easy-to-read format. What I have written may seem like an opinion to some, but I have made the effort to document it. I submit my longevity, of being more than 12 years healthy since being declared free of acute myeloid leukemia by the doctors, 14 years free of multiple myeloma, and more than 23 years since I was first diagnosed with a plasma cytoma, as an example of what is possible when Western medicine integrates with a "wholistic" approach to living and health care.

I feel that to thoroughly appreciate life and live it confidently, we must believe we are here for a purpose and that we are more than a body. Living is more than just showing up, accumulating stuff, propagating, and then saying, "Thank you very much" or cursing it as it comes to an end. This is where the big "WHY," and answering it for yourself, becomes valuable. My family was all I needed as a reminder. I needed to see those little boys become young men. I must be there for my sons and for Beth; I wanted to experience having a rewarding marriage together. What is your big "WHY?"

This journey has strengthened my belief that we did not develop into incredible adaptive organisms by happenstance, and that there is a loving, universal intelligence in our design. I'm not sure, nor am I concerned about, what name anyone wants to give this entity. I just know I've experienced moments of crazy, unrealistic coincidences following prayers and meditation—little voices within or vivid dreams that were answers to personal struggles. Or a person came into my life at the right time, possibly saving my life. Random possibilities, maybe, but it has happened so many times that it seems unlikely.

Through my efforts, I discovered just how amazing the human body, and its complexity, really is. The communication with specific areas of the brain and how much it has to fit in place in order for you to function and survive is awe inspiring. The immune system is so complex, as if a committee of mechanical, electrical, chemical, computer, and even civil engineers designed it, constantly asking, "What if...? Then what?" It is a synergistic operation combining collective functions of bodily systems to address a myriad of concerns. All by chance?

There needs to be increased emphasis placed on the concept of self-care, physically, emotionally, and mentally; together, they create a synergy for good health. Learning to live by the idea, I am "*respondible*" to life by my choices, is incredibly empowering. Feeling a sense of power in your thinking and purpose can lead you to important self-care and choices.

Success in any endeavor is about our focus on personal power and directing our concentration to the things most satisfying to us. This idea brings to mind a quote by Oliver Wendell Holmes: "Many people die with their music still in them. Too often, it is because they are always getting ready to live. Before they know it, time runs out." When I was diagnosed with multiple myeloma, I believed I still had music in me; "songs" I wanted to share. What about you? Which of your songs have gone unsung?

My driving desire and the reason for publishing this book is the hope that maybe my experiences will encourage others not to let cancer, or any struggle, take away the music still within. Your greatest gifts or talents can be mostly celebrated when you use them to help yourself and others to enjoy life more, assisting in expanding and flourishing and increasing joy.

The saying goes, and I paraphrase, "It's not the destination but the journey that matters."

Although I believe the *Journey* statement has truth at its core, an interpretation of this proclamation I once heard to be most relevant is more in line with, "It's who you become on your journey that matters." And having a definite purpose motivates us to start and prevail.

Sir Edmund Hillary and his Sherpa Tenzing Norgoys, the first persons to scale Mount Everest, would have been unsuccessful if they had just decided to go for a nature walk, without a determination to make it to the top. Yet, the persons they became during each of their climbing expeditions, including prior failed attempts at Everest, forged their determination to be triumphant in summiting the top of the world.

Cancer is our Everest. The desire to win is essential, but defining winning is significant. Stay focused on the intention of the desired outcome. For some, it may be to live long enough to realize specific milestones, such as a daughter marrying or a son's graduation. Or perhaps it's to live with cancer while controlling it, as is recognized with less aggressive types of prostate cancer. If being cancer free is the aim, knowing the quest to achieve it and not letting cancer "have you," as defined earlier, is to be victorious.

Made in the USA
Columbia, SC
05 July 2025